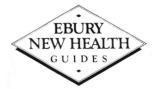

EBURY
NEW HEALTH
GUIDES

D0676201

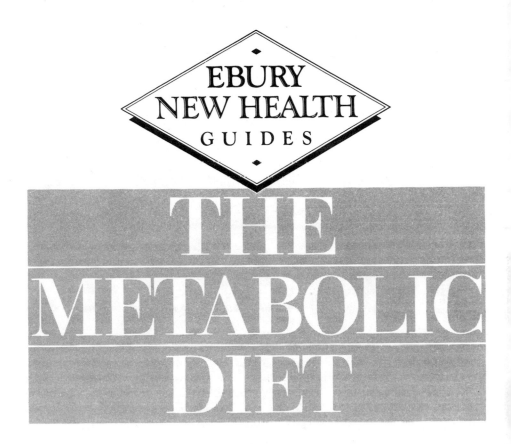

EBURY NEW HEALTH GUIDES

THE METABOLIC DIET

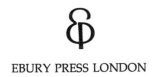

EBURY PRESS LONDON

PATRICK HOLFORD

Published by Ebury Press
Division of The National Magazine Company Ltd
Colquhoun House
27–37 Broadwick Street
London W1V 1FR

First edition 1987
Reprinted 1989

ISBN 0 85223 566 6

Edited by Mike Franklin
Designed by Peter Bridgewater Associates
Computerset in Great Britain by
ECM Ltd, London
Printed and bound in Great Britain by
The Bath Press

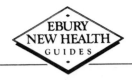

EBURY
NEW HEALTH
GUIDES

CONTENTS

INTRODUCTION   6

DIETING DOESN'T WORK   9

WHY THE METABOLIC DIET WORKS   14

FACTOR 1 – THE VITAMIN FACTOR   20

FACTOR 2 – THE METABOLIC DIET   26

FACTOR 3 – GLUCOMANNAN FIBRE   40

FACTOR 4 – THE BLISSS EXERCISES   45

THE METABOLIC DIET   58

METABOLIC SUPPLEMENTS   69

MONITORING YOUR FITNESS AND FATLESSNESS   71

METABOLIC RECIPES   75

WORK OUT YOUR OWN METABOLIC DIET   100

BINGEING – THE ALLERGY CONNECTION   121

INDEX   126

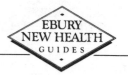

INTRODUCTION

M OST diets say that what you eat, less what you 'burn off' through exercise, ends up as a wadge of fat around your middle. The only way to slim is to eat less or exercise more. But why do some people eat masses and never seem to put on weight, while others have to survive off almost nothing to avoid the pounds creeping on? And why is it that fat people actually eat less food per pound of bodyweight than thin people? The difference is the key to weight loss without starvation. The difference is metabolism.

WHAT IS METABOLISM?

In a very real sense, you are what you eat, because the protein foods that you eat are broken down and reconstituted into your body cells. Carbohydrate-rich foods, like bread or sugar, are necessary to give us energy, as are fatty foods, but when we eat too many fats or carbohydrates the excess turns to body fat. This process of turning food into energy is called metabolism. The more energy you can get from food the faster your metabolic rate. People with fast metabolisms usually have lots of energy, often eat a lot, but never seem to put on weight. It's as if they have a fast-burning 'food stove' that needs constant stoking. Overweight people tend to have a slow metabolic rate. Their slow-burning fire needs only the occasional morsel to keep it going, and consequently they have less energy and have to watch what they eat.

HOW TO RAISE YOUR METABOLIC RATE

The importance of raising metabolic rate has been known for many years to be the most effective way of losing weight. By taking amphetamine-based 'slimming pills' or by drinking gallons of coffee your metabolism will speed up and the pounds will drop off – but not without serious side-effects. Apart from the health risks that these approaches entail, they also lower your metabolic rate when you stop the treatment. They are not a long-term answer to weight loss.

This book tells you how to raise your metabolic rate, which is the only way to stay permanently slim without continually dieting, or becoming a professional athlete. What's more, the only side-effects you are likely to experience are increased vitality, better sleeping patterns, improved digestion and a sharper memory. It is based on four proven factors that help to raise metabolism and keep it balanced.

1 The Vitality Diet

The Vitality Diet is not based on counting calories. It's a diet that ensures that all the food you eat contains the maximum amount of nutrients needed to metabolize it quickly and efficiently. The Vitality Diet improves the efficiency of the body, helping to balance and improve metabolic rate.

2 The Vitamin Factor

However, diet alone is not enough. Many vitamins, and also minerals, are needed for proper metabolism. Taken as supplements, a special combination of vital nutrients helps to boost metabolic rate and assist weight loss.

3 Glucomannan Fibre

One of the keys to balancing metabolism is to prevent rapid increases or drops in levels of sugar (which is what all carbohydrate food breaks down to) in the bloodstream. Rapid changes can result in increased appetite and food cravings, and conversion of sugar to fat. That's where glucomannan fibre comes in. Unlike ordinary fibre, glucomannan fibre helps to stabilize blood sugar levels, reducing appetite and balancing metabolic rate.

4 The BLISSS Exercises

The BLISSS exercise programme is a simple check to see whether the exercise you do maximizes your metabolic rate. If you don't do much exercise, the BLISSS exercise programme will help you to get started. As little as 15 minutes exercise three times a week is enough to make a difference to your metabolic rate.

THE METABOLIC DIET IS EASY TO FOLLOW

Unlike many diets, the Metabolic Diet is not difficult. In fact, many of our clients who have succeeded in losing weight this way have said how much they enjoy the diet and how surprised they were to lose weight without apparently eating any less.

Rosemary, for example, weighed 10 st and wanted to weigh 9 st. And four months later she did. At her follow-up consultation she said, 'I've been on diets all my life. I found losing weight on this diet surprisingly easy. I thought Christmas would be difficult, but it wasn't. I don't want to eat as I did before.'

Hilary lost 2 st 8 lb over six months, and with it she lost her low energy, her pre-menstrual problems, her frequent headaches and bad skin. Like most of my clients, she found the diet remarkably easy. And like almost all my clients her loss of weight and well-being were still improving one year later.

LONG-TERM RESULTS, NOT SHORT-TERM MIRACLES

But don't expect to lose a stone in a month. Instant weight loss usually means long-term weight gain, because dieting actually slows down your metabolic rate. In fact, your metabolic rate can drop by as much as 40 per cent on a crash diet. Perhaps this is why so many of the Weight-watchers Slimmers of the Year are back to the same weight one year later. It is much better to lose a pound a week, and keep it off, rather than a pound a day and put it back on. After all, even a pound a week means you can lose a stone in under four months. If you've spent years putting it on, don't expect fat to go away in a matter of days.

In Part 1 of the Metabolic Diet the facts behind each factor are explained in detail. By understanding the principles behind the Metabolic Diet, it will make it easier for you to pinpoint which factor is most important for you and help you to succeed in losing weight.

Part 2 tells you exactly what you need to know and do to start the Metabolic Diet today. But first of all, let's take a look at why many diets don't work – at least in the long run.

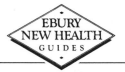

CHAPTER 1

DIETING DOESN'T WORK

A RMED with calorie charts and even calorie calculators countless people have performed mathematical equations over breakfast, lunch and dinner. Although the most popular approach to weight loss, calorie counting is not without its difficulties, nor its failures. We decided to test the practical usefulness of this approach by asking ten long-term overweight women to follow a 1,000 calorie diet (including high fibre foods) for a period of three months. All the women had been overweight for many years and were clearly committed to completing this diet. They were given diet sheets and recipes. Six out of the ten dropped out before three months and reverted to their usual eating habits. These are the results of those four who stuck to their diets as best they could.

Person	Weight Before	Weight After	Loss in lb
1	186	171	15
2	142	146	−4 (Gain)
3	189	187	2
4	156	156	0

Average weight at start was 12 st (168.25 lb)
Average weight at finish was 11 st 11 lb (165 lb)
Average loss in weight was 3.25 lb.

Calorie counting worked for one out of four who said they completed the three-month diet, but worked for only one in ten who started the diet with good intentions. Many dieters will blame themselves. 'The diet works but I don't. I have no will-power. If only I stuck to the diet better and for longer. Next time . . .' and the pounds creep back on. Yet there is some truth to this. The support of slimming groups and coercion of the weight-loss clubs may increase that iron will we're meant to have. But what is the point of recommending a diet that few can stick to?

A calorie is a unit of energy. Technically, a calorie is the amount of heat needed to raise one gram of water by one degree Centigrade. The dieter's calorie is actually a kilo-calorie (a thousand calories). The calorie content in food varies according to the type of food. Fat is most calorific, followed by carbohydrate then protein. On the other side of the balance, different activities use up different amounts of calories. For example, an hour of walking uses up 200 calories, while half an hour of energetic cycling may use up 250 calories. If you eat more than you burn off in activity you get fat, and if you eat less than you burn off you get thin. Simple isn't it?

THE CON BEHIND CALORIE COUNTING

According to Dr Colgan, author of *Your Personal Vitamin Profile*, some of the athletes he works with burn off over 7,000 calories, but eat only 3,500 calories. By calorie theory, these athletes should have disappeared completely by now. An investigation by Dr Apfelbaum of people living in famine in the Warsaw ghetto during the second world war shows the same contradiction. With an average calorie intake of 700–800 calories per day, and a daily requirement of say 2,500 calories, a deficit of 1,241,000 calories would build up over two years. The average body has 30 pounds of fat, representing 100,000 calories, to dispose of. Even if all this fat were lost, what happened to the remaining one million calories?

Since one pound of fat is roughly equivalent to 4,000 calories, eating 40,000 calories less per year would mean losing 10 lb in the first year, $3\frac{1}{2}$ st by the fifth year, over 7 st by the tenth year and vanish entirely after 15 years! All by eating one less apple every day. Because one apple provides 100 calories a day or 36,500 a year. Turn the equation round the other way, and the simple sin of an extra daily apple would mean a gain of 7 st every ten years.

The calorie equation for exercise is equally ridiculous. Cycle vigorously for 15 minutes each day and you will lose 10 lb in the first year – quite possibly, but 7 st after ten years? No chance. However, according to calorie theory, one apple a day undoes all that hard work.

The problems with calorie theory are not just mathematical ones. Proponents of calorie theory, like Audrey Eyton, author of *The F-Plan Diet*, have realized that the major problem to calorie controlled diets is that people get hungry. The question became 'How can we eat 1,000 calories a day and feel satisfied?' The answer was fibre.

THE FIBRE FAD

Within days of publication of *The F-Plan Diet*, fibre sales had exploded. My wife Liz, who runs a health shop, was ordering bran in 5 foot sacks, and selling it faster than she could pack it in bags. This by-product of refining flour had been promoted to a princely food, but partly for the wrong reason. Studies using increased quantities of grain fibre do not consistently report effects on weight. Now, although the fibre boom still continues, many have found that high fibre, low calorie diets are not the mecca they had hoped. With this boom came high fibre tablets and high fibre convenience foods promoted as the slimmer's best friend.

The table below shows the results of such a diet, with a recommended intake of 35 g of fibre per day. The results are not impressive. We further tested high fibre tablets without a calorie controlled diet. Again we took ten overweight women and put them on either Vita Fiber or Slim Aide tablets. Each Vita Fiber tablet contained 500 mg of cereal fibre. Slim Aide, on the other hand, contained only 100 mg of cereal fibre. Each participant received six tablets a day, which was the manufacturer's recommended dose. Five out of ten dropped out, and these are the results of the remaining five three months later.

Person	Weight Before	Weight After	Loss in lb
1 (SA)	144	140	4
2 (SA)	158	151	7
3 (VF)	119	122	−3 *(Gain)*
4 (VF)	198	198	0
5 (VF)	196	196	0

(VF = VITA FIBER, SA = SLIM AIDE)

Average weight at start was 11 st 9 lb (163 lb)
Average weight at finish was 11 st 7 lb (161.4 lb)
Those on Vita Fiber gained on average 1 lb
Those on Slim Aide lost on average 5 lb

Neither the effect of these high fibre tablets nor the effect of a high fibre diet appears to be great, although they may help a small percentage of people. However, high fibre diets are definitely recommended for many other health reasons. For instance, it is well known that those on high fibre diets have less risk of bowel cancer, diabetes, or diverticular disease, and are unlikely to suffer from constipation.

Fibre is a natural constituent of a healthy diet high in fruits, vegetables, nuts, seeds and grains. There is no need to add extra bran if these foods are eaten. Professor Dickerson from the Nutrition Department at the University of Surrey has stressed the danger of adding bran to a nutrient-poor diet, since bran contains a high level of phytate, which reduces our absorption of some essential minerals, including zinc. I never recommend bran without ensuring adequate zinc status.

Fibre is calorie free and there is little doubt that a diet high in fibre is more satisfying and easier to follow. After all, which would you find easier to eat: two sweet biscuits, or a pound of carrots?

While we have learned that low calorie diets do help maintain correct weight and that high fibre content in the diet makes this easier, there are many more pieces of the jigsaw.

EAT FAT, GROW SLIM?

Advocates of high-fat, low carbohydrate diets believe that if you don't eat carbohydrate you must burn fat instead. Fat is, after all, a very good form of fuel, giving twice as much energy per gram. But burning fat is a bit like lighting a log with a match – it doesn't work. You need kindling to get a good 'fat' fire burning and carbohydrate is the kindling. So just like a fire that smokes because it burns inefficiently, a high fat diet gives off smoke in the form of 'ketones'. High-fat theorists claim that this inefficient metabolism means a loss of potential fat calories as ketones are excreted. But other scientists beg to differ. Research has clearly established that, at most, 100 to 150 kcal are lost in ketone excretion and, what is more worrying, excessive ketone levels are extremely dangerous.

HIGH PROTEIN DIETS

High protein, low carbohydrate diets are also to be avoided for health reasons. By restricting carbohydrate intake, inefficient fat breakdown may occur, again causing an increase in ketones. Protein may also be used for fuel, and the advocates of this approach argue that protein is hard to convert and therefore less calories are consumed by the body at the end of the day. There may be an element of truth in this, but any diet which aims to imbalance metabolism is at best a short-term answer and at worst positively bad for your health. After all, 58 deaths have been associated with low calorie, high protein diets.

FASTING DIETS

Modified fasts are the most severe approach to dieting. For those with life-threatening obesity they may be of value, but they are certainly not for the average person. One study followed 207 patients hospitalized for fasting over nine years. While 79 reduced their weight to within 30 per cent of their ideal weight, 90 per cent of these were back to their original weight nine years later. Hardly a long-term solution.

STARCH BLOCKERS DON'T WORK

'Just swallow these pills and they'll stop you digesting starch, so you can eat as much as you like without getting fat.' That was the argument put forward in 1983 when sales of starch blocker tablets rocketed throughout the world. Dr Hollenbeck studied the effects of these starch blockers and found no evidence of any effect on carbohydrate metabolism. They also found very variable levels of the starch enzyme inhibitor, as well as lectin which is a potentially dangerous substance in beans, from which the raw material was derived. Lectin is destroyed in cooking. The only significant physiological changes these pills had was an increase in flatulence! So watch out for Jack and his magic beans.

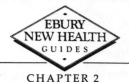
CHAPTER 2

WHY THE METABOLIC DIET WORKS

THE principle behind the Metabolic Diet is plain common sense. By increasing your metabolic rate and changing your diet so you're eating more in quantity but a little less in calories the net effect has to be weight loss. To understand how to increase your metabolism you need to understand how metabolism works.

Everything you eat (except vitamins and minerals) can be divided into fat, protein or carbohydrate. All of these can be converted by the body into glucose (sugar) and from there, into fat or energy. This transition happens through a series of chemical reactions, activated by enzymes, which are dependent upon different vitamins and minerals. But not all types of food are easy to convert into energy. Some require more energy to initiate the chemical reactions than others.

1 g of FAT *gives 9 kcal of energy*
1 g of PROTEIN *gives 4 kcal of energy*
1 g of CARBOHYDRATE *gives 3.75 kcal of energy*

Fat gives more energy per gram than protein, and is therefore more calorific. That's the energy equation. What about the health equation?

PROTEIN

Protein is what you are made of. Twenty-five per cent of you is protein. Your hair, nails, skin and bones are all protein. Protein is made up of smaller units called amino acids. Each protein has at least 20 amino acids arranged in a distinct order. Amino acids are like the letters of the alphabet, and each protein is like a word. Countless different words can be made from 26 letters of the alphabet and so it is with protein. That's what makes the difference between skin or nails, or rabbit protein and human protein. Ideally, we eat protein for one reason only – that is to replace old body cells. We don't need it for energy. Carbohydrates are our most ideal fuel. Too much protein is hard work for the body to eliminate.

FAT

But if fat provides more calories, surely it's a better energy source than carbohydrate? If our bodies were simply energy machines this would be true, but they're not and too much fat has its problems. First of all, since fat is higher in calories it's easier to eat more of it and put on weight. What's more, the higher the level of fat circulating in your bloodstream, the greater the risk for heart disease, diabetes and kidney disease to start with. Too much fat means the body has to break it down and get rid of the excess. There are a number of stages that can go wrong, and the result may be extra work for the kidneys or a build-up of fats in the blood and in the artery walls.

But fat is not all bad. Some fats, called essential fatty acids (EFAs), are like vitamins. We've got to get them, otherwise we get ill. These EFAs are found mainly in the leaves and seeds of plants, and are also high in fish. We also need some fat to help absorb the fat-soluble vitamins. The fat on our bodies, which acts as padding, can be made from dietary fat or carbohydrates.

HOW FOOD TURNS INTO ENERGY

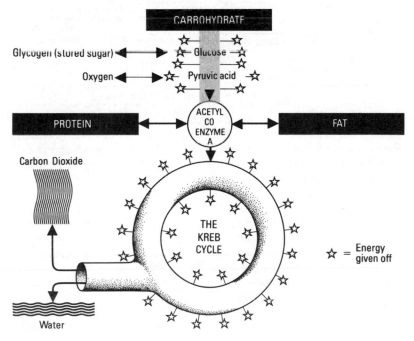

CARBOHYDRATES

Carbohydrates are the best kind of energy food. A carbohydrate, for example potato, is broken down through a series of chemical reactions, the end product being glucose, which is the simplest carbohydrate called a sugar. This takes place over a matter of hours and provides us with a gradual supply of energy. You might think then why not just eat glucose, or other simple sugars like sucrose (white table sugar), fructose (fruit sugar) or dextrose?

FAMILY TREE OF CARBOHYDRATES

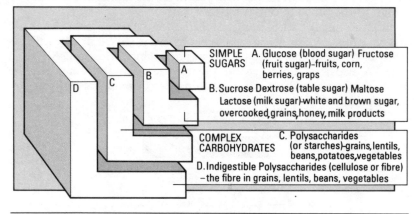

SIMPLE SUGARS A. Glucose (blood sugar) Fructose (fruit sugar)–fruits, corn, berries, graps

B. Sucrose Dextrose (table sugar) Maltose Lactose (milk sugar)–white and brown sugar, overcooked grains, honey, milk products

COMPLEX CARBOHYDRATES C. Polysaccharides (or starches)–grains, lentils, beans, potatoes, vegetables

D. Indigestible Polysaccharides (cellulose or fibre) – the fibre in grains, lentils, beans, vegetables

THE SUGAR BALANCE

It's all a question of balance. First of all, maintaining an even blood sugar level is probably the most crucial factor in our body chemistry. Rapid changes cause all sorts of problems from food cravings to depression. The early warning signs are usually mental or emotional imbalances because when we're not exercising, the brain uses half of all the energy expenditure of the body, despite the fact that 50 per cent of our weight is muscle and only three and a half pounds are brain.

Secondly, our bodies are designed to slowly break down complex sugars through a series of enzyme reactions, each controlled in sequence. Just eating sugar disturbs this sequence and metabolism becomes inefficient. And lastly and most importantly, complex carbohydrates contain the vitamins and minerals needed to metabolize them properly. Simple sugar does not.

Let's take a closer look at the importance of blood sugar levels. When we eat sugar it passes through the wall of the digestive tract and enters the bloodstream. Naturally, the blood sugar level rises. This rise tells the body that it needs to lower it and help get the sugar to the cells to be used for energy or put into storage. This is achieved by a very special chemical called insulin, which is produced in the pancreas. Insulin helps to carry the sugar to the cells and as it does this, the blood sugar level drops down again to the normal level and everything is balanced. At least, that's what is meant to happen.

In reality, one in ten of us are 'glucose intolerant' which means we have a less than perfect control of blood sugar. Fat people are particularly likely to be glucose intolerant. Here's what can go wrong.

The blood sugar can rise too rapidly, for too long, without being checked by insulin. This results in high blood sugar. Then when the insulin is released, too much can be released and the blood sugar level goes too low, too fast. This is known as hypoglycaemia (hypo = low; glyc = glucose; aemia = in the blood). Another common cause of glucose intolerance is a deficiency of the mineral chromium. Insulin cannot work properly without chromium, so although the insulin may be released it doesn't have much effect. In the advanced stages of diabetes the body may have completely lost the ability to produce insulin.

THE SUGAR CYCLE

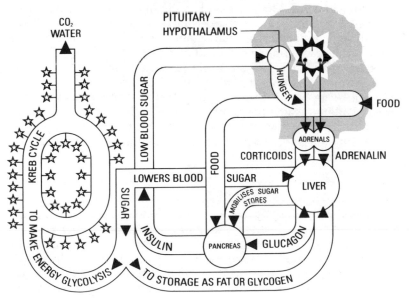

Any one of these problems will result in glucose intolerance and there are many symptoms associated with this problem. These include irritability, aggressive outbursts, nervousness, depression, crying spells, vertigo and dizziness, fears and anxiety, confusion, forgetfulness, inability to concentrate, fatigue, insomnia, headaches, palpitations, muscle cramps, excess sweating, digestive problems, allergies, blurred vision, lack of sex drive and excessive thirst. Do any of these sound like someone you know?

STIMULANTS ACT LIKE SUGAR

But not only sugar can cause these problems. So can stimulants like too much tea and coffee. Stress, whether that means rows at home or pressure at work, has exactly the same effect. Because all stimulants, whether nutritional or emotional, set up a chain of reactions that push up our blood sugar level. To understand why this happens we need to take a look at our ancestors.

Cavemen or monkeys need energy when under stress, because the only stresses in nature are hunting, fighting or being hunted. The stress of hunger and the thrill of hunting for food triggered the chain of reactions that released stores of glucose, vital for clearer brain function and active muscles. Modern man has the same chemistry but a very different world. Shopping in a supermarket can hardly be described as hunting and, under normal circumstances, you don't have to compete with your fellow shoppers for a loaf of bread.

Modern-day stress is more likely to come from problems within relationships, pressures at work, financial commitments, or from the stress of being bored. Unconsciously there's a part of us that loves stress. Children watch horror films and play Space Invaders. Adults watch 'thrillers' or contact sports, or take part in dangerous pursuits from skiing to fast driving. Others turn to stimulants like cigarettes, coffee, tea and sugar.

THE STRESS REACTION

Any form of stress will raise your blood sugar level. This happens immediately because stress stimulates the release of the powerful hormone adrenalin. Adrenalin stimulates the liver to release stored sugar. It makes your heart beat faster and your blood vessels constrict to get the sugar to the cells extra quick. It heals wounds fast – and eventually it slows down your metabolism. It's funny to think that, even as you sit impatiently in a traffic jam, your blood is coagulating because your body hears STRESS = FIGHT = HEAL WOUNDS FAST.

Adrenalin also tells the liver to release the hormone glucagon, which in turn is a powerful stimulator of insulin release from the liver. In prolonged stress this adrenal reaction is maintained by the adrenal hormone called corticosteroids (cortisone is a corticosteroid).

REGULATING YOUR APPETITE

When your blood sugar level is low this makes you feel hungry. The low sugar level actually stimulates a portion of the brain called the hypothalamus, which increases your appetite. Sudden drops in blood sugar level, which can occur only minutes after food if you are glucose intolerant, and more normally occur three hours later, can lead to ravenous appetites which sometimes start off bingeing.

It is well known that fat people are less responsive to the increased rise in blood sugar so they may just keep eating without hearing the body signals to stop. For this reason small, frequent meals are best.

Once the blood sugar has returned to normal and glucose has left the bloodstream there is still a long way to go before energy is produced. The extraction of energy from glucose takes place in every cell in the body. Muscles need energy to work, new cells need energy to be built, and nerve cells need energy to pass along their messages. And most importantly, the brain needs energy, which is why glucose intolerance results in disturbed mood and mental performance.

No less than 13 vitamins and minerals are needed to make this last stage work, and only if these are optimally supplied is metabolism most efficient. That's the first key to the success of the Metabolic Diet. The Vitamin Factor.

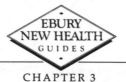

CHAPTER 3

FACTOR 1
THE VITAMIN
FACTOR

You can't live without vitamins and minerals. Even though we need only tiny quantities weighing less than a hundredth of the amount of protein we need they are just as important. And you can't maintain an even metabolism and stay healthy without them.

But, can't you get all you need from eating a well-balanced diet? That depends what you mean by 'need'. If all you 'need' is to be averagely healthy and averagely fat then the answer is probably yes. But if you want to be super healthy and stay the right weight without having to worry about what you eat, getting your optimum levels of vitamins and minerals is the place to start.

In one survey, the diets of 100 health-conscious people were analysed. Only 32 had a diet that conformed to the current standards set for a 'well-balanced diet'. From these 32, no less than 24 had multiple symptoms of vitamin and mineral deficiency. And these findings are nothing new. In 1981 a survey by the Bateman Catering Organization reported that 'more than 85 per cent of the women and their families ate a diet which did not provide the daily nutrient intakes recommended by the DHSS.' They also found that, when interviewed, these women thought they were already eating a 'well-balanced diet'.

OPTIMUM NUTRIENT RANGE

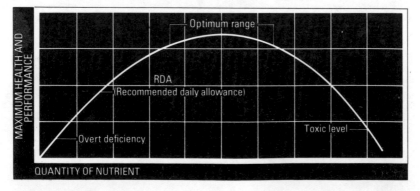

The difference between obtaining the basic nutrient requirements and the optimum nutrient requirement may be the difference between moderate health and excellent health, or overweight and perfect weight. The graph on page 20 shows how physical performance and health increase, until a certain point where performance may decrease as the nutrient dosage continues.

YOUR PERSONAL VITAMIN PROGRAMME

The levels of nutrients you need to provide optimum nutritional support are dependent on a wealth of factors, some seemingly unconnected with nutrition. To arrive at the most suitable nutrition programme all these should be carefully evaluated. The eight factors we assess are as follows, although it should be pointed out that, as time goes on, this list will grow and our means for evaluation will become more accurate.

1 Hereditary Factors

Optimum nutrition is different for every one of us. No two people ever have the same energy requirements. Just as no two people ever look the same. Our nutrient needs, like our looks, are dependent on our parents and grandparents. Small nutrient deficiencies in our ancestors may mean increased nutrient needs in us. For instance, a study by Lucille Hurley at the University of California induced a short-term zinc deficiency in a group of pregnant rats. Their offspring showed weakened immune systems (associated with zinc deficiency) despite having good zinc status all their lives. Their offspring's offspring also had poor immune function and so did their offspring's offspring's offspring – all because of a transient zinc deficiency three generations earlier! So the first rule of nutrition is to pick good parents.

2 Biochemical Individuality

No two children born of the same parents, exposed to the same environment, will have identical nutritional needs, even though we would expect them to be close.

Whatever the circumstances, every individual is unique. Each person's biochemical uniqueness must be assessed in building an optimum nutrient programme. Professor Roger Williams from the University of Texas has established the scientific fact of biochemical individuality, both for animals and humans. Vast differences in organ size, enzyme production and subsequently in nutrient needs are commonly found. Tenfold differences in nutrient requirements are not uncommon, although threefold differences are more usual. Therefore it is vital to measure biochemical function – through biochemical tests and/or sub-clinical symptoms and not just through dietary analysis.

3 Current and Past Nutrient Intake

Minor deficiencies in diet will manifest as sub-optimum symptoms like poor memory, poor dream recall, poor nail and hair condition, or simply a lack of energy. Usually the first symptoms of a poor diet affect mental ability as our brain is perhaps our most delicate and carefully balanced organ. By following the vitality diet a number of dietary deficiencies can be avoided. However, it is not only what you eat that is important but also where it is grown.

Mineral deficiencies vary from country to country depending on the soil levels. For instance, many northern hemisphere countries, including Britain, are low in selenium, zinc and manganese. This may be due to glaciation in the past, and over-farming in the present. Even the best organically grown vegetables are only as good as the soil they are grown in.

4 Current and Past Anti-Nutrient Intake

An anti-nutrient is a substance which interferes with the action of a nutrient, either by preventing its absorption, disturbing its chemical utilization, or by promoting its excretion. Toxic metals like lead and copper are good examples of anti-nutrients which interfere with zinc and calcium utilization. Many natural foods contain small amounts of anti-nutrients. For example, wheat contains phytates which interfere with zinc absorption. An excessive consumption of wholemeal bread can seriously deplete zinc levels.

Some 2,000 chemical additives are used in food production, many of which act as anti-nutrients. Some of these are not easily excreted from the body, so past intake of these and other anti-nutrients must also be assessed.

5 Absorption

For some nutrients, as little as 5 per cent of the amount supplied from the diet can actually be absorbed. Only a third of the calcium supplied in the diet is actually absorbed. This tends to be the rule, not the exception, and it exemplifies the importance of proper enzyme levels and healthy intestines to ensure maximum absorption. There are many reasons for malabsorption of nutrients ranging from physical problems like a faulty ileo-caecal valve, to chemical problems like poor hydrochloric acid production in the stomach. If absorption is poor this must be corrected before vitamin supplements can be properly utilized.

6 Stress Level

Stress is not an easy word to define, as it involves both the situations we are in and the way we react to those situations. Either way, too much work and too little sleep puts a strain on our bodies which subsequently use up more energy, and demand more nutrients. Stress includes the mental and emotional components of our lives, which are equally subject to pressure and imbalance. When these areas of our lives create stress, simply improving one's nutrition will not solve any problems. However, it is said that the body is the temple of the soul – and you can't build a temple out of sugar.

7 Use of Stimulants and Drugs

Like stress, adrenal stimulants use up more energy and deplete us of nutrients. So do substances like alcohol and some medical drugs which tax the body's detoxifying mechanisms. Adrenal stimulants include tea, coffee, sugar, salt and cigarettes.

8 Exercise

Exercise is the single most important factor that alters our overall nutritional requirements, other than our age. An athlete in training may expend four times as many calories of energy as a person leading a sedentary lifestyle. Clearly, such an athlete would have very different nutritional needs.

To obtain the best (and quickest) results all these factors should be taken into account in building your ideal nutrient programme. While some people respond within a month, it is wise to expect it to be three months before you feel substantially different.

VITAL VITAMINS FOR REDUCING WEIGHT

Twenty-two vitamins and minerals are needed for proper metabolism and weight control. Although our needs vary from person to person, ten of these are vital for improving metabolism and helping to break down fat. These are vitamins B1, B2, B3, pantothenic acid, B6, C, choline, inositol, chromium and zinc. This is what the most important ones do:

B6 is fundamental for the production of pancreatic enzymes, which ensure smooth digestion. It is also needed for the production and regulation of sex hormones and adrenalin and helps produce brain chemicals involved with our moods. B6 is best taken with zinc. 100 mg to 300 mg of B6 per day is recommended.

B3 (nicotinic acid) is one of the constituents of GTF (Glucose Tolerance Factor, see Chromium) needed to maintain our blood sugar balance. It is essential for converting unused glucose to glycogen, the body's short-term reservoir of energy. In doses of 1 g B3 lowers cholesterol levels. Normally 50 to 250 mg per day is quite adequate.

Vitamin C has many roles to play in weight control. Firstly, it is needed for hormone production in the adrenal glands and is a vital link to preventing glandular exhaustion leading to slow metabolism. It is involved in the conversion of glucose to energy in the cell. Like B3 it also lowers elevated cholesterol levels. The recommended daily dose is 1 to 3 g.

Chromium is the major nutrient in GTF released every time our blood sugar level rises. GTF makes insulin more effective and is therefore crucial for balanced blood sugar levels. Chromium is widely deficient, especially among the elderly. 20 to 100 mcg is recommended daily.

Zinc is probably the most deficient mineral in Britain. It is involved in over 20 different enzyme reactions, including the energy cycle. Zinc deficiency disturbs sense of taste and smell, as well as appetite. Deficiency of zinc is also associated with stretch marks, poor wound healing, poor eyesight and may be involved in anorexia nervosa and bulimia. In case you're wondering, becoming zinc deficient is not the way to lose weight! 15 to 25 mg is needed each day. But the average diet provides only 11 mg and even less if you're a vegetarian.

These nutrients need to be supplemented every day, together with a good multivitamin and multimineral supplement to provide the other important micronutrients. The chart on page 25 lists my closest approximation to the ideal levels of vitamins and minerals to be supplemented daily on top of the Metabolic Diet (Chapter 4) for the 'average' person.

Vitamin	Optimum Daily Level	Mineral	Optimum Daily Level
Vitamin A (retinol)	7,500 iu	Calcium	200 mg
Vitamin B1 (thiamine)	75 mg	Magnesium	100 mg
Vitamin B2 (riboflavin)	75 mg	Iron	12 mg
Vitamin B3 (niacinamide)	175 mg	Zinc	17.5 mg
Vitamin B5 (pantothenate)	75 mg	Manganese	6 mg
Vitamin B6 (pyridoxine)	175 mg	Chromium	120 mcg
Vitamin B12 (cobalamine)	10 mcg		
Folic Acid	100 mcg		
Choline	50 mg		
Inositol	50 mg		
Vitamin C (ascorbate)	2,000 mg		
Vitamin D	400 iu		
Vitamin E (d-alpha tocopherol)	100 iu		

The following list of supplements meets these needs:

Supplement	AM	PM
Vitamin C 1,000 mg	1	1
Multivitamin	1	
B Complex	1	
B6 100 mg+Zinc 10 mg		1
B3 100 mg+Chromium 100 mcg	1	

These supplements are best taken 15 minutes before, after or during a meal. Do be careful to check the dosage carefully, as well as the price, when buying supplements. Good brands are: Healthcrafts, Meadowcroft, Quest, Cantassium and Health+Plus. This programme will cost around 40p a day. The benefits are far more than just weight loss.

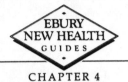

CHAPTER 4

FACTOR 2
THE METABOLIC
DIET

IT isn't just the quantity, but the quality of what you eat that makes the difference to your weight and health. Different foods have quite different effects on metabolism, depending on the type of fat or sugar they contain, whether they're rich in the right vitamins or minerals, their fibre content and a host of other vital factors. In fact, there are five important qualities within your diet and these form the five key principles of the Metabolic Diet.

THE FIVE KEY PRINCIPLES

1 The Well-balanced Diet

Everybody talks about it, but few of us really know what a well-balanced diet is and how to get it. Using a new and simple system called the Batterham Diet Balancer, which is explained in Part 2, you can work out simply and accurately just how well balanced your diet is. You'll be surprised to find out which foods are high in fat, and how a few simple changes to your diet and favourite recipes can give you a diet balanced for protein, carbohydrate and fat content.

2 The Vitamin Vitality Diet

The Metabolic Diet recommends foods that are high in vitamins and minerals, since these are the cornerstones of a well-balanced body chemistry. But these essential micronutrients are not only missing in most over-processed foods, but are also destroyed by over-cooking. So the Metabolic Diet gives you hot and cold recipes that involve the minimum of cooking – and time!

3 Special Food Factors and Fibre

It used to be thought that only one kind of fibre counted. That was cellulose, or indigestible carbohydrate. But recent breakthroughs in nutrition have identified special plant proteins and fats that help maintain even levels of circulating fat and sugar. This diet takes these special food factors into account.

4 Balancing Blood Sugar

Keeping a stable blood sugar level is perhaps the most vital key to efficient metabolism and appetite control. When the blood sugar level is out of balance hunger pangs and food craving develop. But not all foods that contain carbohydrate, which breaks down to sugar, have the same effect on blood sugar. Certain types of carbohydrate-rich foods have less dramatic effects on blood sugar. These are used in preference in the Metabolic Diet.

5 Stimulant Free Diet

Like sugar, excesses of coffee, or any other stimulant, will also alter the blood sugar level and hence the metabolism. The Metabolic Diet is therefore a low stimulant diet. But let's start at the beginning.

BALANCING YOUR DIET FOR FAT, PROTEIN AND CARBOHYDRATE

Most of us eat a diet that is far too high in fat and sugar. This is more likely to make us overweight and unhealthy for two reasons. The first is that too much fat simply isn't good for you. It increases the risk for heart disease, cancer, diabetes, gall bladder and kidney disease. Since most fat comes from eating too much meat, cheese or eggs, we can also get more protein than we need. The net result is no appetite for carbohydrates, like vegetables, beans, grains and even fruits.

The recommended levels of these macronutrients are 30 per cent of our calories from fat, 15 per cent from protein, 55 per cent from complex carbohydrate. The 'average' person eats 40 per cent fat, 15–20 per cent protein and 45–50 per cent carbohydrate, one-third of which comes from sugar, and up to a quarter from alcohol. However, according to a survey by the Bateman Catering Organisation the large majority of us think we are eating a well-balanced diet. When interviewed, only one in ten people who said they ate a balanced diet actually knew what a well-balanced diet was. The big problem is not so much what we are eating, but knowing what we are eating so something can be done!

The Batterham Diet Balancer is an ingenious solution to this problem. It is a very simple system for looking at your diet and working out in a minute whether or not your meal is balanced. Each meal is calculated to contain a certain number of Fat Points, Protein Points and Carbohydrate Points. If these points are balanced your diet is balanced. If not, it's easy to see why not.

For example, two slices of bacon and a fried egg gives 195 Protein Points, no Carbohydrate Points, and 215 Fat Points. Given that you only need 300 points of each for the day, this common breakfast has already provided two-thirds of all protein and fat needed for the day, and is disastrously deficient in complex carbohydrates.

Take another example – baked beans on two slices of wholemeal toast, with a small amount of butter. This provides 85 Protein Points, 60 Carbohydrate Points and 45 Fat Points. The figures are much more balanced and so is this meal. The fat level is down, but notice how easy it is to get enough protein without eating meat.

In Part 2 you'll find 30 days of 'points balanced' menus to get you started on the Metabolic Diet. There's also a chapter to show you how to work out your own balanced diet. After a while, you can forget about the charts and the menus because you'll just know when your diet is right.

VITAMIN VITALITY

Nature often supplies foods together with their complement of the vitamins and minerals needed to metabolize them properly. Due to over-farming, over-cooking and most of all, over-processing, many of the foods that make up a typical Western diet are sadly deficient in vitamins and minerals. For example, refining sugar, flour or rice removes over 92 per cent of the mineral chromium, essential for helping insulin to work.

MINERAL LOSSES IN REFINED FOOD			
	White Flour	Sugar	White Rice
Chromium	98%	95%	92%
Zinc	78%	88%	54%
Manganese	86%	89%	75%

Modern farmers have learnt how to over-farm their land by adding fertilizers like NPK. The short-term result is more crops and more profits. But the plants become mineral deficient as the soil gets depleted and unable to take up what minerals are left due to the chemical effect of the fertilizers. It is not surprising to find that some oranges, when analyzed, are found to contain no vitamin C: that spinach, supposedly an excellent source of iron, can contain from

0.1 mg to 138 mg per 100 g, depending on where it is grown. Once more, it is we who are short changed and the result is compromised nutrition and subsequently less than perfect health and metabolism.

So which foods have vitamin vitality? Dr Roger Williams from the University of Texas devised an excellent way to measure and see at a glance the vitamin vitality in foods using a chart system.

Each chart shows a sphere with thin lines, like spokes on a wheel, each representing one essential nutrient. These are subdivided into *Amino Acids, Vitamins, Major Minerals, Trace Minerals* and *Others*. The first chart shows thick lines extending to an inner circle. This represents a fictitious diet that would supply exactly the recommended daily levels of each nutrient. The next chart shows the average British diet. Those thick lines which don't reach the inner circle represent a nutrient frequently shown to be deficient.

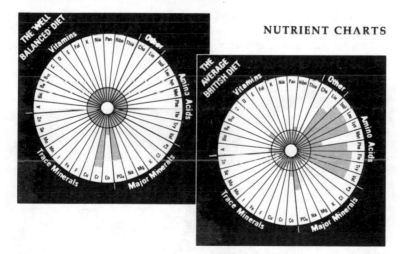

NUTRIENT CHARTS

As much as two-thirds of the average calorie intake is fat, sugar and refined flours. These are called empty calories because they provide no nutrients. Often hidden in processed foods and snacks, they usually weigh less and instantly satisfy our appetite. For instance, two sweet biscuits provide more calories than a pound of carrots and are considerably easier to eat – but they provide no vitamins or minerals. If a quarter of your diet, by weight, and two-thirds by calories, is such dismembered foods, there's little room left to get adequate levels of the 39 essential nutrients.

NUTRIENT CHARTS

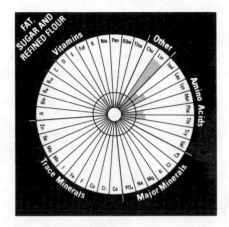

Wheat, for example, has 25 nutrients removed in the refining process to white flour, yet only four (iron, B1, B2, B3) are replaced. On average, 87 per cent of the vital minerals zinc, chromium and magnesium are lost. Have we been short changed?

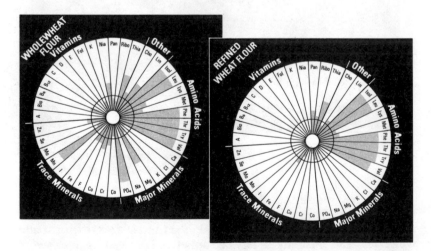

Processed meats like hamburgers and sausages are no better. The use of inferior meat with a high fat content lowers nutrient content. Eggs, fish and chicken are nutrient rich sources of protein. However, as these charts show, protein deficiency is rarely the problem.

NUTRIENT CHARTS

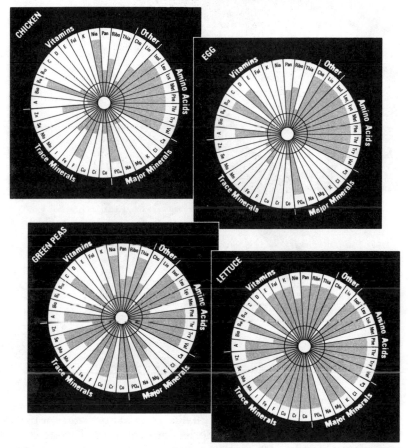

Vegetables, fruits, nuts and seeds are full of vitality. Tomatoes and lettuce, for example, are packed with vitamins and minerals. If anyone says they're just water, remember, even Maggie Thatcher is 65 per cent water! The humble potato is also vitality rich (even though a Birds Eye survey found that more people thought ice cream was good for them than potato!), but make sure you eat them with their skins on. Other fantastic foods are peas (the vegetarian's best source of manganese), bananas (high in potassium), mushrooms, spinach and other green leafy vegetables, as well as beans, nuts and lentils. These foods should make up at least half your diet.

NUTRIENT CHARTS

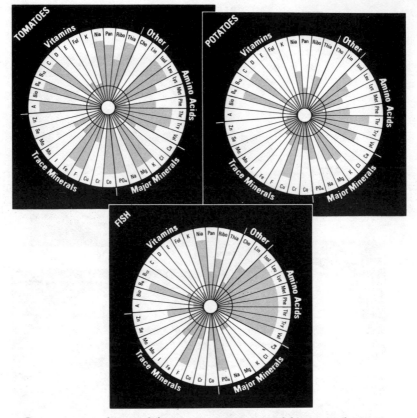

One secret to longer life, greater energy and less weight is to eat foods high in vitamin and mineral quality, high in fibre, and low in fat. Such a diet will also be low in calories, but you don't have to count them. By following such a regime, the body becomes increasingly efficient and does not crave extra food. Craving for food, despite having eaten enough calories, is often a craving for more nutrients. So foods providing 'empty calories' are to be strictly avoided.

SPECIAL KINDS OF FIBRE

There are many different kinds of fibre other than those found on the husks of grains, like wheat bran or oat bran. While these may be best for promoting regularity, 'gum' fibres like pectin (high in apples, carrots and bananas), guar or glucomannan appear to be best for controlling blood sugar levels. Glucomannan, the most effective in clinical trials, is recommended as part of the Metabolic Diet. Foods rich in pectin are also included.

PLANT POWER

But it isn't just fibre that has this effect, according to new work by Drs Story and Thompson in the US. Polyphenols, special ingredients found in beans, have been shown to cause a slower release of sugar into the blood. It is thought that this might explain why diabetics, placed on a diet high in beans, appear to need less insulin. Another substance, this time a group of plant fats called 'saponins', have been demonstrated to keep down blood cholesterol levels, thus reducing risk for heart disease. Saponins are particularly high in unrefined nuts and seeds, and especially alfalfa sprouts or seeds. All these beneficial foods are used liberally in the Metabolic Diet. But now it is time to turn our attention to foods that are not beneficial to our metabolism. And top of the list is sugar.

IMPROVING GLUCOSE TOLERANCE

Glucose is the simplest chemical form of sugar. All the carbohydrate (sugar and starch) we eat is broken down into glucose or fructose – the only forms in which it can be absorbed by the body and turned into energy. This glucose enters the bloodstream as soon as digestion is complete. Normally, the pancreas then reacts by producing insulin, which takes the glucose out of the blood and into the cells.

WHAT GOES WRONG?

If we constantly eat sugar, the pancreas can become over-stimulated. If we eat any carbohydrate in refined form (white sugar, sweets, chocolate, white flour) digestion is rapid, and glucose enters the blood in a violent rush. In each case, the pancreas can over-react and produce too much insulin. Blood glucose then takes a rapid, uncomfortable drop – and may end up too low for normal functioning. When this is pronounced this is called hypoglycaemia (hypo = low; glyc = sugar; aemia = in the blood). If this over-stimulation happens too often, the pancreas becomes exhausted. Now, instead of too much insulin it produces too little. Too much glucose remains in the blood (hyperglycaemia). In its most severe form, this condition becomes diabetes.

GLUCOSE INTOLERANCE

The regulation of blood glucose is a constant balancing act. The aim is to provide energy to the cells which need it (especially the brain), and to make sure that unwanted glucose is not left circulating in the blood.

RESPONSES TO GLUCOSE

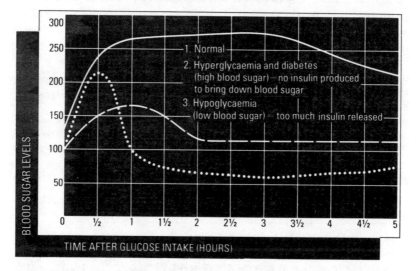

1. Normal
2. Hyperglycaemia and diabetes (high blood sugar) — no insulin produced to bring down blood sugar
3. Hypoglycaemia (low blood sugar) — too much insulin released

BLOOD SUGAR LEVELS

TIME AFTER GLUCOSE INTAKE (HOURS)

If this balance is lost, both physical and mental well-being are, in turn, unbalanced. Low blood glucose (hypoglycaemia) and high blood glucose (hyperglycaemia) can have similar and wide-ranging effects: irritability, aggressive outbursts, nervousness, depression, crying spells, vertigo and dizziness, fears and anxiety, confusion, forgetfulness, inability to concentrate, fatigue, insomnia, headaches, palpitations, muscle cramps, excess sweating, digestive problems, allergies, blurred vision, excessive thirst and lack of sex drive. Do any of these sound like someone you know? All these symptoms have been noted in people with glucose intolerance.

For most people glucose intolerance will correct itself in time, if the diet is changed to exclude stimulants and refined sugar. Stress too can play a large part. Vitamins (especially B and C) give important support to the adrenal glands while things get back to normal. And the mineral chromium is important in the formation of glucose tolerance factor (GTF), a substance released by the liver which makes insulin more potent.

THE STRESS REACTION

STRESS FACTORS
job pressure, anxiety, shock, lack of sleep, salt, sugar,
cigarettes, alcohol, coffee, tea, horror films, electronic games . . .

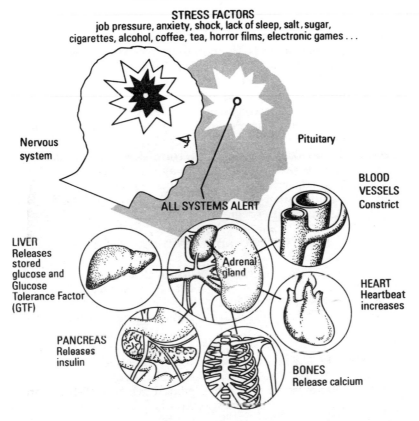

Nervous system

Pituitary

ALL SYSTEMS ALERT

BLOOD VESSELS Constrict

LIVER Releases stored glucose and Glucose Tolerance Factor (GTF)

Adrenal gland

HEART Heartbeat increases

PANCREAS Releases insulin

BONES Release calcium

Here are some other helpful hints if you think glucose intolerance may be part of your problem. Eat small, frequent meals, preferably containing protein. Always eat breakfast. Avoid sugar, and foods containing sugar. Dilute fruit juice with water. Avoid convenience foods or foods containing long lists of preservatives as they are almost certain to contain refined carbohydrates and various harmful chemicals. Decrease your intake of dried fruit. Decrease your intake of alcohol. Drink less tea and coffee. Decaffeinated coffee is also best reduced, as it still contains other stimulants.

STABILIZING BLOOD SUGAR LEVEL

With the right diet, your blood sugar level should become more stable, like graph 3 in the figure above. Using these blood sugar curves, Dr

Jenkins and his colleagues set out to find which foods had the greatest effect on blood sugar levels. He measured the space under the curve, calling this the glycaemic index. Foods with a high 'glycaemic index' had the most drastic effect on blood sugar. His results, shown below, were not quite what you would expect.

Grains had a small effect on blood sugar level, but when grains were refined the effect became greater. Rice went from 66 to 72 when refined. The best grains in this test were buckwheat and wholewheat spaghetti. Of the breakfast cereals tested, cornflakes came out the worst and porridge oats the best by a long way. Oat cakes also have little effect on blood sugar. Many root vegetables, particularly carrots and potato, had a surprisingly large effect on blood sugar. This effect may be very dependent on the degree of cooking.

THE GLYCAEMIC INDEX OF COMMON FOODS

Grain, cereal products

Bread (white)	69
Bread (wholemeal)	72
Buckwheat	51
Millet	71
Pastry	59
Rice (brown)	66
Rice (white)	72
Spaghetti (wholemeal)	42
Spaghetti (white)	50
Sweetcorn	59

Dried legumes

Beans (tinned, baked)	40
Beans (butter)	36
Beans (haricot)	31
Beans (kidney)	29
Beans (soya)	15
Beans (tinned, soya)	14
Peas (blackeye)	33
Peas (chick)	36
Peanuts	13
Lentils	29

Breakfast cereals

All-bran	52
Cornflakes	80
Muesli	66
Porridge oats	49
Shredded wheat	67
Weetabix	75

Fruit

Apples	39
Bananas	62
Oranges	40
Orange juice	46
Raisins	64

Biscuits

Digestive	59
Oatmeal	54
Rich tea	55
Ryvita	69

Dairy products

Ice-cream	36
Milk (skimmed)	32
Milk (whole)	34
Yoghurt	36

Vegetables		Sugars	
Broad beans	79	Fructose	20
Frozen peas	51	Glucose	100
		Maltose	105
Root vegetables		Sucrose	59
Beetroot	64	Honey	87
Carrots	92	Mars Bars	68
Parsnips	97	Lucozade	95
Potato (instant)	80		
Potato (new)	70		
Swede	72		
Yam	51		

The best foods from all those tests were pulses – peas, beans and lentils. None of these had a substantial effect on blood sugar. Milk products which contain the sugar lactose were also good. Surprisingly, even ice-cream came out well. But don't kid yourself – it's still high in fat and sugar, even if it doesn't alter blood sugar level much.

Fruits, being high in fruit sugar, had quite a strong effect on blood sugar. Raisins, being concentrated, were the worst with bananas a close second. Apples were the best. But fruit sugar, fructose, has much less of an effect than glucose or maltose. Sucrose, which is table sugar, is a combination of glucose and fructose and was in between these two for its glycaemic rating. Very high up the list are Lucozade, Mars Bars and even honey. Despite some interesting findings the overall effect is clear. Any form of concentrated sugar affects blood sugar balance.

YOU DON'T NEED EXTRA STIMULATION ON THIS DIET!

Stimulants act much like sugar, since they cause blood sugar levels to rise, as the adrenal glands stimulate the liver to release glycogen stores. Stimulants include tea, coffee, chocolate, cola drinks, cigarettes, some medications and, although not strictly stimulants, salt and alcohol are included because these do affect the adrenal glands and glucose balance in the body.

You don't need to avoid all of these all the time, but it is worth knowing that their drug-like effect on the body may sometimes provide short-term lifts in mood and energy, but in the long run excessive use of stimulants is no cure for obesity. So what do they do?

Alcohol is made by the action of yeast on sugar. As such it has a similar action on glucose metabolism as sugar. Alcohol inhibits the release of reserve glucose from the liver and depresses the demand for more sugar by the hypothalamus, thus contributing to low blood sugar problems and increased appetite. Alcohol interferes with zinc absorption, and increases the absorption of lead. Excessive consumption greatly increases the risk for diabetes, heart disease, cirrhosis and cancer of the liver.

Chocolate contains cocoa as its major 'active' ingredient. Cocoa provides significant quantities of the stimulant theobromine, whose action is similar to although not as strong as caffeine. Theobromine is also obtained in cocoa drinks, like hot chocolate.

Cigarettes contain nicotine as well as 16 cancer producing chemicals. Nicotine is the primary stimulant and has a substantial effect in very small dosages. In large amounts nicotine acts as a sedative. The individual variation in reaction to nicotine is considerable. A recent medical report on addictive drugs lists nicotine as more addictive than heroin. People breaking the habit often experience extreme low blood sugar problems.

Coffee contains theobromine, theophylline and caffeine, all of which act as stimulants. Caffeine is the major stimulant. A cup of coffee contains about 60 mg. However, decaffeinated coffee still provides theobromine and theophylline. Theophylline disturbs normal sleep patterns. Coffee consumption is associated with greater risk for cancer of the pancreas, and during pregnancy is associated with an increased incidence of birth defects. Children consuming excess caffeine become hyperactive. Withdrawal from caffeine can result in headaches, which subside after four days.

Cola drinks contain between 5 and 7 mg of caffeine which is a quarter of that found in a weak cup of coffee. In addition, these drinks are often high in sugar and colourings and their net stimulant effect can be considerable.

Food Colourings, particularly azo dyes, of which tartrazine (E102) is one, have a stimulant effect on sensitive individuals and have been clearly linked with hyperactivity in children.

Medications provided for the relief of headaches may contain caffeine. Other caffeine tablets are available as stimulants. The most common are Pro Plus and the herb Guarana.

Salt contains sodium which acts as an adrenal stimulant causing a diuretic effect. Excess sodium also raises blood pressure. Sodium is mildly addictive. Excessive salt consumption is often associated with loss of sense of taste or smell caused by zinc deficiency. No added salt is needed for good health.

Tea contains caffeine, theobromine and theophylline. It is a stimulant and a diuretic with similar, although diminished effects of coffee. A very strong cup of tea can provide as much caffeine as a weak cup of coffee. Tannic acid present in tea interferes with the absorption of many important minerals. Tea drinkers have an increased risk for stomach ulcers.

The Metabolic Diet detailed in Chapter 7 takes into account all these key principles to give you a diet which balances and improves metabolism. Although you may not think so when you eat the delicious recipes, it is a proven diet for losing weight – without any side-effects except increased health and vitality.

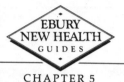

CHAPTER 5

FACTOR 3 GLUCOMANNAN FIBRE

THE high fibre approach has a number of good points. Firstly, a shift to high fibre foods, basically wholegrains, fruits and raw vegetables, is a shift to a healthier nutritious diet. A diet high in fibre is also known to protect against diseases of the colon, especially cancer, as well as cardiovascular disease. A high fibre diet is also more satisfying. After all, most of us could eat two bars of chocolate, but what about 5 lb of carrots?

What the F-Plan Diet ignores is the fact that there are many different forms of fibre, with different effects on weight loss. One of these is Glucomannan. Glucomannan, unlike many fibres which make up the outside shell of a plant cell, is found within the plant cell of the Japanese 'Konjac' plant. The Konjac plant (whose Latin name, *Amorphophallus*, gives you an idea of what it looks like!) has been grown and used as food for years by the Japanese. My attention was drawn to this unusual fibre by two studies reporting astounding weight loss with only 3 g of Glucomannan a day. (Most weight loss diets recommend at least 35 g of fibre per day for any effect.) One study at the University of California gave 12 obese people 3 g of Glucomannan per day and found an average weight loss of 9.7 lb. David Walsh at the GNC research centre replicated this study over a four-week period under double-blind conditions and found a 5.3 lb weight loss.

These stories sounded too good to be true. Slimming without suffering! Just take a few pills each day and the pounds will drop off AND you get healthier – because Glucomannan has some very beneficial side effects. It decreases the diabetic's need for insulin, it lowers the levels of triglycerides in the blood, which are associated with heart disease, and is a very effective cure for constipation.

We decided to test this 'wonderfibre' for ourselves. We selected 40 obese women and assigned them to one of four groups. Group A received placebos (dummy tablets); group B received tablets containing 500 mg of pure Glucomannan; group C received Vita Fiber, or Slim Aide, two top-selling slimming tablets based on ordinary grain fibre and group D went on a calorie controlled diet using supplementary placebos. To make sure the test was fair we matched the groups for average weight, which was 12 st 2 lb. The experimenter who interviewed the participants was instructed to read out a speech explaining when and how to take the tablets, and that they were a new form of fibre. Each participant received the same speech and neither they nor the experimenter knew that dummy tablets and different forms of fibre were being used. Three months later we analysed the results.

Not only did those on Glucomannan lose a substantial amount of weight, without any alteration to diet and exercise, but their weight loss was significantly better than those following a calorie controlled diet, or taking other 'hi-fibre' tablets. Those on the dummy tablets lost no weight, so we knew the Glucomannan effect was real. The table below shows the individual's loss in weight. This varied from a loss of 16 lb to a gain of 2 lb, with an average weight loss of 6.6 lb.

Subject	Weight Before	Weight After	Loss in lb
1	140	136	4
2	194	196	−2
3	271	267	4
4	147	141	6
5	181	183	−2
6	168	155	13
7	189	173	16
8	162	154	8
9	185	174	11

Average weight before = 13 st (182 lb)
Average weight afterwards = 12 st 7 lb (175.4 lb)
Average weight lost = 6.6 lb

The surprising results of Glucomannan alone illustrated to us just how different 'fibres' can be. Since Glucomannan swells to 100 times its original volume when placed in liquid, we wondered whether its effect in weight loss was due to decrease in appetite caused by swelling in the stomach. Wheat bran, which only swells to three times its volume, may have been ineffective for this reason. However, only two out of nine women on Glucomannan experienced any suppression or reduction of appetite. In the placebo group, one out of three did, and one out of five did in those taking other high fibre tablets. Although Glucomannan may slightly suppress the appetite, it is unlikely that this is the major reason for its success. Glucomannan does prevent extreme overeating and in that respect would be useful to those who binge.

GLUCOMANNAN REDUCES HEART DISEASE

Glucomannan's first appearance in medical journals was not as a slimming aid, but as a powerful reducer of cholesterol and triglycerides in the blood. These fats are strongly associated with cardiovascular disease, as is excess weight itself, and much medical research has focused on drugs and natural substances for reducing these blood lipids. Much of the work has been carried out in Japan, although some studies have been done in America. Studies by Kishida 1969, Inhami 1973, Tsuji 1975, Nagai 1978, Oku 1981 and Walsh have all shown Glucomannan to be a reliable reducer of high blood cholesterol and triglyceride levels. For example, Kishida gave three patients with elevated blood cholesterol levels 3 g of Glucomannan each day and noted a significant reduction in cholesterol levels. He then tested this anti-cholesterol effect by administering 70 g of butter in the diet and increasing the dose of Glucomannan to 12 g. Once more, blood cholesterol levels declined.

Glucomannan appears to block, to some extent, the absorption of fat and cholesterol and this is almost certainly a factor in its effective use in weight loss. Dr David Walsh from the Research Department of GNC in America found the same results. When he studied 18 patients with cholesterol levels ranging from normal to high, he found a significant reduction over an eight-week period while on Glucomannan.

These results indicate the importance of fibre, and especially Glucomannan fibre for maintaining a healthy heart and circulatory system.

GLUCOMANNAN AND DIABETES

Another fascinating area of Glucomannan research has been in the field of diabetes. Diabetics are unable to properly control the level of glucose (sugar) in their bloodstream, primarily due to a poor production of insulin. Insulin is produced by the pancreas and, when released into the bloodstream, helps transport glucose to the cells. Most diabetics have impaired insulin production and subsequently suffer from the effects of high blood sugar.

Dr Matsuura from Kobe University, Japan, investigated the role

Glucomannan has for stabilizing blood sugar. Initially, he had found that supplementing 2.6 g of Glucomannan before giving the patient an intake of glucose, significantly delayed and reduced the rapid rise in blood sugar level. This suggested that Glucomannan successfully delays the absorption of glucose, as has been shown with other dietary fibres.

He then supplemented 13 diabetics with 3.9 and 7.8 g of Glucomannan per day for 90 days. After 20 days their cholesterol level had dropped by 11.2 per cent and their fasting glucose level by 29 per cent after 30 days. This allowed him to reduce the therapeutic dose of insulin or other glucose lowering agents, and in some cases insulin treatment was stopped altogether.

Guar gum, another form of dietary fibre, has for some time been known to have this effect. Therefore a comparison of these two was the next step for clinical research. It has now been confirmed that Glucomannan reliably lowers fasting glucose level and is more effective than any other dietary fibre tested to date.

This is of far reaching importance for those with weight problems, as obesity and diabetes are closely related. Many obese people are diabetic and, of those who are not, many are unable to maintain the appropriate blood glucose levels, resulting in glucose intolerance. This is called hypoglycaemia when the blood sugar level goes below a certain level and hyperglycaemia or diabetes when the glucose level rises too high. Both are more likely to occur with people who eat a diet high in refined carbohydrates like sugar and refined flour. Inability to control blood sugar level often leads to binge eating and frequent use of stimulants like coffee, or sugary foods, as an attempt to get energy by raising the blood sugar level. Glucomannan fibre provides an effective way out of this vicious circle of food craving.

GLUCOMANNAN RELIEVES CONSTIPATION

Like other dietary fibres, Glucomannan speeds up transit time of food through the intestinal tract by providing bulk. This also has the added advantage of diluting toxic substances in the intestines and rendering them less harmful. However, Glucomannan actually slows down stomach emptying, allowing longer time for digestion and a longer feeling of satiation.

Glucomannan has been tried and tested as a natural means for relieving constipation. The results of Japanese research show that people suffering from chronic constipation respond to only 1 g of

Glucomannan within three days of administration. Therefore Glucomannan is more likely to be used in this respect in the future than other forms of dietary fibre. However, a more long-term approach to constipation is recommended, involving dietary changes and an increase in exercise. Fibre of any sort is only effective if taken on a daily basis. Constipation will soon return when Glucomannan is stopped if one's diet and exercise remain unchanged.

HOW TO TAKE GLUCOMANNAN FIBRE

Unlike other forms of dietary fibre, 3 g of Glucomannan per day is enough to induce weight loss as well as stabilizing blood sugar levels, and lowering cholesterol levels. Since 3 g is approximately a table-spoon of powder, this can be taken in capsule form or made into a gel with water. Either way, Glucomannan should always be taken with a large glass of water, as it is extremely absorbent.

It is best taken 30 minutes before eating in order to obtain the maximum reduction in appetite.

Glucomannan fibre comes in 500 mg capsules, therefore six tablets must be taken each day. If you eat three major meals a day, it is best to take more Glucomannan before the largest meal. For example:

Breakfast	Lunch	Dinner
1 capsule	2 capsules	3 capsules

Some people have experienced slight bloatedness and an increase in intestinal wind for up to seven days after starting Glucomannan. This is the only side effect noted and disappears completely within a week.

Glucomannan Fibre is available from Health+Plus, Quest, Cantassium and Meadowcroft. These are widely available in healthfood shops.

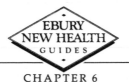

CHAPTER 6

FACTOR 4
THE BLISSS
EXERCISES

THE good news about exercise is that you really don't have to be fanatically fit to lose weight. And the reason why is not calories, it's metabolism.

According to the calorie theory, exercise doesn't do much to promote weight loss. After all, a three mile run only burns up 300 calories. That's equivalent to two slices of toast or a piece of apple pie. But this argument, upon which has hinged the preference to eat less rather than exercise more to lose weight, misses four important facts.

The first is that the effects of exercise are cumulative. OK, so running a mile a day only burns up 300 calories, but if you do that three days a week for a year that's 22,000 calories, equivalent to a weight loss of 11 lb! Also, the amount of calories you burn up depends upon how fat you are to start with, how hard and how long you exercise and how much of you is fat or muscle. For example, consider someone who weighs 14 st compared to someone weighing 9 st. If the 14 st person runs one mile in eight minutes, and the 9 st person does it in ten minutes, the heavier person will use up over 1,000 calories, and the lighter person will only burn up 550 calories. The table overleaf shows how many calories you can use up by running, depending on your weight, distance and speed. An 8 st person, running at five miles per hour for one hour, will use up 405 kcals, while a 16 st person running at ten miles per hour will use up 1,635 kcals – over three times as much.

But if you are overfat and underfit to start with, don't expect immediate results through exercise. The reason is this. Most of us are relatively fit in our school years. School encourages us to play sports and children and adolescents are naturally more physically active. Consequently a larger proportion of younger people is muscle rather than fat. Muscle cells need lots of fuel and therefore burn lots of calories. The leaner the muscle gets the more it needs oxygen. The best kind of exercises are 'aerobic' exercises, which means exercises which supply oxygen. In fact, you can measure how hard a muscle is working by how much oxygen it uses up. Continuous exercises like swimming, jogging or

ENERGY EXPENDITURE DURING A ONE HOUR RUN
(in calories)

Body Weight	MPH	5	6	7	8	9	10
8 stone		405	493	573	655	737	900
9 stone		469	551	643	735	827	920
10 stone		510	611	713	815	917	1020
11 stone		563	675	788	900	1013	1127
12 stone		614	735	858	981	1104	1228
13 stone		663	794	927	1060	1161	1326
14 stone		713	854	997	1139	1282	1426
15 stone		768	919	1074	1227	1381	1536
16 stone		818	980	1143	1307	1471	1635

Adapted from McArdle, W.D. et al Exercise Physiology: Energy, Nutrition and Human Performance. Lea and Febiger, 1981.

cycling are more aerobic than stop-go exercises like tennis or squash. Exercises like squash use more 'fast-twitch' muscle which uses glucose as fuel. Running uses more 'slow-twitch' muscle which uses fat for fuel. You will lose weight playing squash but you have to play it for a long, long time compared to swimming, running or cycling.

So what happens when you leave school, start driving to work rather than walking, and cut down your overall amount of physical activity?

First of all, your good lean muscles start to turn to fat. If you go on a crash diet, your body will break down these good lean muscles to use for energy, and in both cases the result is less muscle. And since muscle uses up calories there is less of you to burn up the food you eat. So putting on weight becomes easier.

As you start to exercise you will begin to replace that fatty muscle with lean muscle and rebuild muscle that you didn't have before. With extra muscle you'll begin to burn off that excess fat faster and faster. So even though you may not lose weight with exercise to begin with you are replacing fat with muscle and becoming less fat, and that's what counts for long-term weight loss.

HOUSEWORK WON'T KEEP YOU FIT

Another myth about exercise is that you can keep fit through housework. So many times I've asked clients how much they exercise only to hear them say 'I don't do exercises as such, but I'm on my feet all day at the office, or running my home.' Old textbooks will tell you that the average houseperson or sedentary worker will burn up 2,500 calories,

HOW TO INCREASE YOUR BASELINE ACTIVITY

The Fat Way	The Fit Way
Take the lift	Use the stairs
Use a trolley when shopping	Use a hand basket
Drive to work	Walk or cycle some of the way
Drive to the shops	Walk to the shops
Buy convenience foods	Cook fresh foods
Spend the night watching TV	Take up an active hobby
Get other people to bring you drinks	Get up and do it yourself (and get them one too!)
Use powered tools for gardening or DIY work	Use manual tools when it's just as quick
Go upstairs as little as possible at home	Run upstairs as often as possible
Use automatic car washes	Wash it yourself
Stick children in front of TV	Actively play with them
Have business meetings inside	Go for a walk where possible.

so by putting people on a 1,750 calorie diet, the net effect should be a substantial weight loss. But new research and improved methods for measuring energy expenditure show that these figures are slight distortions of the truth. In fact, a sedentary worker or houseperson will burn up around 2,000 calories a day. Reducing intake to 1,750 calories a day would not have a substantial effect.

The good news is that you can double your energy output without doing any exercise as such. How? By increasing your baseline level of activity. And that's what the BL stands for in the BLISSS exercise programme. Your baseline activity is the amount of energy you use up just going about your normal life. You can double this in a hundred different ways. For example, use the stairs instead of lifts. Walk the last mile to work. Use a hand basket rather than a trolley in the supermarket. Even chopping vegetables rather than eating already prepared convenience food will give you more exercise! Every little bit counts.

For example, one study examined the effects of walking on six overfat and underfit young men. Five days a week for 16 weeks they walked for 90 minutes a day. That's the equivalent of 45 minutes to work and back. They lost an average of 12.5 lb, their percentage of body fat dropped from 23.5 per cent to 18.6 per cent and their blood fat levels improved, which is a measure of heart health.

That means that if you could walk the last 15 minutes to work and back you would lose 14 lb in a year, without making any extra effort to exercise. The chart on page 47 gives you other ideas for increasing your baseline level of activity.

UNFANATICAL FITNESS DECREASES YOUR APPETITE

Contrary to popular belief, moderate exercise actually decreases your appetite. According to new evidence on appetite research, both animals and man consistently show decreased appetite with small increases in physical activity. One study looked at an industrial population in West Bengal, India. Those doing sedentary work ate more and consequently weighed more than those doing light work. As the level of work increased from light to heavy, workers ate more, but not relative to their energy output. The result was that the heavier the work the lighter the worker.

EFFECT OF EXERCISE ON CALORIC INTAKE AND BODY WEIGHT

Job Classification	Daily Caloric Intake (kcal)	Body Weight (lb)
Sedentary	3,300	148
Light work	2,600	118
Medium work	2,800	114
Heavy work	3,400	113
Very heavy work	3,600	113

It appears that a degree of physical activity is necessary for appetite mechanisms to work properly. Those who do not exercise have exaggerated appetites and hence the pounds gradually creep on. With moderate exercise and the other key factors within the Metabolic Diet, there is no need to go hungry while losing weight.

EXERCISE BOOSTS YOUR METABOLIC RATE

But the most important reason why exercise is a key to weight loss is its effect on your metabolic rate. According to Professor McArdle, exercise physiologist at City University, New York, 'Most people can generate metabolic rates that are eight to ten times above the resting value during sustained running, cycling or swimming. Complementing this increased metabolic rate is the observation that vigorous exercise will raise the metabolic rate for up to 15 hours after exercise.' In fact, other studies have shown that metabolic rate is raised by 25 per cent for 15 hours and by 10 per cent for 48 hours. According to sports physiologist Professor Fenton 'Exercise has a stimulating effect on metabolism which persists throughout the day, raising metabolic rate and leading to the loss of appreciably more fat than would have been predicted for the exercise taken.' The metabolic effect of exercise is far more significant than the calories used up in the exercise itself. Simply by doing 12 minutes of aerobic exercise a day you can substantially increase your metabolic rate, without increasing your appetite. The net result is weight loss.

EXERCISE – HOW TO GET STARTED

The 'I' in the BLISSS exercise programme stands for 'individual', because you as an individual must choose what kind of exercise will be enjoyable for you. The usual mistake that people make when starting an exercise programme is to be over-ambitious. If you're not used to jogging, starting off with a one mile run will overtire your muscles and the last thing you'll want to do the next day is go running. What's more, in the early stages you need as much support as possible. So don't choose solitary sports like jogging unless you're a strong-willed individual.

STARTING AN EXERCISE PROGRAMME

Actually deciding to start an exercise programme is for most people the biggest hurdle to regular exercise. Many runners find it harder to decide to go running, get their shoes on and go out of the front door than the actual run itself. However, once decided upon, there are still a number of other barriers that can prevent the unsuspecting from making their programme a 'programme for life'. Ignorance of the way the mind and body can adjust to exercise and the way it can't, is probably the most important of these barriers. There are three principles which, if understood and followed, can prevent many of the common mistakes that occur as one embarks on a new programme.

THE THREE P PRINCIPLES

Patience

Health or fitness cannot be developed overnight. Many people lose interest in exercise because their bodies do not adapt quickly enough and they are not aware that changes are taking place. Both exercise and weight reduction follow two important rules.

The first is that change doesn't happen overnight. In fact, if you notice a change in either your fitness or your weight from day to day you are probably changing too fast for your body to be able to adapt. The second rule is that your health won't improve from one day's exercise or one day's dieting. The beneficial effects are cumulative, and can only be judged over a period of months, not days. So be patient.

Progression

Few people apply the progression principle to optimum effect. Many start with an excess of enthusiasm and a lack of patience and begin at a level that places excessive stress on the body. This usually results in pain or exhaustion, evaporated enthusiasm and a high drop-out rate.

One of the most important aspects of a good exercise programme is the sense of achievement derived from gradual but continuous improvement. By starting at a level within one's capacity and gradually stretching your capacity without overdoing it, pain, exhaustion and boredom can be avoided.

Perseverance

Ideally, exercise should become an enjoyable habit that fits into your daily routine and is something to look forward to, not an obligation. This does not mean that every training session will be an enjoyable experience. Initial sessions will probably be uncomfortable as the body adjusts to something new. After adaptation has occurred some sessions will still be less enjoyable than others due to a whole variety of reasons. So you need a degree of perseverance.

Not all forms of exercise will help you to lose weight. Some exercises, like weight lifting, develop plenty of strength but have a negligible effect on metabolic rate. Other exercises, for example yoga, develop suppleness, but once again don't change your metabolic rate. It's the endurance exercises that develop stamina and have the greatest effect on speeding up weight loss. The best exercise programmes contain all these three 'S factors' – Strength, Suppleness and Stamina, with an emphasis on stamina.

STAMINA

Stamina or endurance is the ability to perform moderate intensity exercise for a long time without becoming exhausted or out of breath. Stamina exercises develop the heart, lungs and circulation system and so reduce the chance of heart or circulatory disease. For this reason, from a health point of view, this is the most important aspect of exercise.

Stamina exercises are called 'aerobic' exercises because the muscles need a good supply of oxygen as well as glucose to work for any length of time. Short sprints are 'anaerobic' because the body can produce a small amount of energy without oxygen. Long runs become more anaerobic if you push yourself beyond the limit. However, if you run too slowly, the body doesn't have to work hard enough to increase the supply of oxygen to the muscles. And it's the muscles' ability to use up more oxygen that makes your metabolism speed up.

So how do you know when you are exercising aerobically? The secret is your pulse rate. If your pulse increases to the right level, which is explained later, and you keep exercising at this level for a significant length of time, the exercise is aerobic. Swimming, running, walking, skipping, aerobics or dance classes are all forms of aerobic exercise and will help you to lose weight.

STRENGTH

Strength training for health differs considerably from strength training for fitness. An athlete aiming for maximum strength will spend many hours lifting weights, which can result in a very well developed muscular body. In our technology- and machine-based society super strength has become a somewhat redundant asset.

However, strength-promoting exercises can have considerable health-promoting qualities that do not result in excessive muscular development. The body is a rigid skeleton supported by many muscles held in tension. If some of these muscles are too weak or antagonistic pairs of muscles are out of balance, then poor posture can result. Hiatus hernia is an example of a medical disorder that is completely preventable by regularly exercising one's abdominal muscles. Also, strength promoting exercises do convert fatty muscle to lean muscle, helping the muscle to burn fat more efficiently. Since muscles take up less space than fat, strengthening exercises, like weight training or Lotte Berk classes, help you to lose inches faster than pounds.

SUPPLENESS

Suppleness or flexibility is a measure of the maximum range of movement we have in our joints and muscles. Suppleness declines with age more rapidly than any other factor, so maintaining flexibility is a vital component for an active old age. Regular muscle stretching can also reduce stiffness, prevent aches and pains in the muscles, and reduce the chance of injury brought on by vigorous exercise. Thus a stretching routine should be incorporated into your exercise programme.

Contrary to much public opinion, doing stretching exercises by jerking (eg fast repetitions of toe touching, or similar exercises) does not promote maximum range of movement, and increases the risk of injury. Muscles have a stretch reflex which causes the muscles to contract when they are quickly stretched to their maximum limit. Using body weight or momentum to override this safety mechanism can lead to muscle damage. The best way to overcome this is to very slowly stretch to one's mobility limit and then hold the stretch for six to eight seconds. Having adjusted to this limit the muscles relax and loosen and permit you to take the stretch a little further. In this way muscles can be stretched to their full limit and maximum range of movement developed. Yoga exercises incorporate slow stretches and provide an excellent way to promote maximum muscle suppleness and range of movement.

Aerobics and dance classes have grown in popularity in recent years and attempt to combine continuous vigorous aerobic exercise with stretching exercises. As is often the case with combinations of this kind, compromise is necessary in both areas. It is very difficult to produce a sequence of varied exercises for a class of different people that's right for everybody. The speed at which the stretches are performed may also be too fast to allow the stretch reflex to adjust. Nevertheless, the aim of a good exercise programme is fun and enjoyment and many people do thoroughly enjoy their aerobic class. The above warnings are not meant to put people off, but to make them aware of the potential problems that can occur in aerobics classes, taught by inexperienced teachers. A good warm-up is essential, and it is important to ensure that the pace at which the exercises are carried out is not too fast for your body rhythm.

Neither strength nor suppleness exercises can directly result in any significant weight loss. This can only be achieved through raising the metabolic rate so more energy is expended. Aerobic exercise is undoubtedly the most efficient way to achieve this.

CHOOSING YOUR EXERCISE

Exercise	Average time a week to maintain fitness	Stamina rating	Suppleness rating	Strength rating
OUTDOOR				
Running	45 mins	•••••	•	••
Cycling	3 hrs	•••••	••	••••
Hill walking	3 hrs	••••	•	••
Football	3 hrs	•••	•••	••••
Skiing	4 hrs	••	•••	•••
Tennis	5 hrs	••	•••	•••
Golf	8 rounds	••	••	•
Hard gardening	6 hrs	•••	••	•••
INDOOR				
Aerobics (hard)	1 hr	•••••	•••••	•••
Skipping	1 hr 15 mins	•••••	••	••
Dance exercises	1 hr 30 mins	••••	•••••	••
Aerobics (average)	1 hr 30 mins	••••	•••••	••
Circuit training	1 hr 40 mins	•••••	••••	•••••
Swimming	2 hrs	•••••	•••••	•••••
Squash	3 hrs	•••	••••	•••
Psychocalisthenics	3 hrs	••••	•••••	•••
Badminton	5 hrs	•••	•••	••

RUNNING

Running is the quickest method of attaining the minimum level of aerobic fitness and the fitness benefits of running translate well into other sports. Running is accessible and economical – the only real necessity being a pair of good quality running shoes. On the minus side running can become boring if done alone. Also, it has no effect on exercising the upper body and injuries are very common in running, especially running on hard surfaces. The impact of each jogging step is two to three times bodyweight. Knee injuries are the most common followed by injuries to the lower legs and feet. These potential problems can be overcome by investing in top quality running shoes.

ROPE SKIPPING

Skipping is accessible, very economical and is a very effective method of attaining aerobic fitness. An all-weather activity, skipping also works the upper body to some extent and develops co-ordination. Skipping is not recommended if you are very overweight as excess strain will result on knees, ankles, lower back etc. and injury could result. Skipping for 20 mins or so continuously also involves a certain amount of skill and many people lack the co-ordination necessary.

CYCLING

Cycling is accessible, relatively economical, and is a good way of acquiring aerobic fitness. Although it requires two to three times as much time as running per week to obtain fitness, cycling is preferable for overweight people as there is no strain on the joints and cycling is often a more enjoyable introduction to exercise for sedentary people.

SWIMMING

Swimming is an excellent all round activity which develops strength and flexibility as well as stamina. It is relatively cheap and accessible and as the bodyweight is supported by the water there is no strain on the weight-bearing joints, making it an ideal activity for overweight people. It is often difficult however to swim continuously for 30 minutes or more in crowded public baths.

TENNIS

Tennis is essentially an intermittent (non-continuous) activity and therefore has to be played for a long time to gain any aerobic benefit. Tennis is a very enjoyable activity and it is probably advisable to get fit to play tennis rather than use tennis as a means of becoming fit.

CIRCUIT WEIGHT TRAINING

Circuit weight training consists of a routine of exercises for acquiring aerobic fitness and muscular strength and endurance. The abundance of fitness centres makes this relatively accessible and economical. Circuit weight training should be performed under the guidance of a qualified instructor. It may be too strenuous for the very overweight who should acquire a base level of aerobic fitness via a different activity (walking, cycling, etc.) before starting circuit weight training.

WALKING

Walking is an excellent first aerobic exercise for the previously sedentary person. However, the walking needs to be vigorous and involve a few hills to provide good exercise.

SQUASH/BASKETBALL/FOOTBALL

As with tennis these are intermittent sports demanding shorter bursts of more concentrated activity. Squash, in particular, is too strenuous a game to be used by the overweight person to acquire fitness. As before, it is advisable to get fit to enjoy these sports rather than use the sport to become fit.

MONITORING YOUR FITNESS

For maximum metabolic effect, whatever exercise you choose it should be sufficiently hard to raise your pulse rate to 80 per cent of its maximum. If you exercise too hard the heart will have to pump too fast and your muscles may not get enough oxygen. This will overtire your muscles and get you nowhere. On the other hand, if you don't work hard enough it may take you half an hour before you reach the ideal pulse rate for increasing your metabolism.

Your maximum heart rate depends on how efficient your heart is. A young person's heart may have a maximum rate of 200 beats per minute, while a person over 40 would be very unwise to exceed a pulse rate of 180. The chart below shows you what your maximum heart rate is, depending on your age. The pulse rate you should be aiming for in exercise is 80 per cent, unless you have a history of heart disease, in which case even this may be too high. While many recovery clinics for heart disease patients recommend not exceeding 75 per cent, it is wise to check with your doctor first.

TAKING YOUR PULSE

Your pulse can be found inside the bony protuberance of the thumb side of your wrist. Alternatively, you can take it by placing your fingertips on the side of your neck. You will, of course, need a watch with a second hand. Normally, for medical examinations your pulse is taken for 30 or 60 seconds, but to find your pulse while exercising, stopping for this long would lower your pulse and give you a false reading. So for our purposes, your exercise pulse whould be taken for six seconds only, immediately on stopping your exercise, then multiply the result by ten. This gives you your exercising pulse. To begin with you may need to stop briefly every five minutes to monitor your pulse, but after a while just measuring it at the end of your exercise session will suffice.

YOUR IDEAL AEROBIC PULSE RATE

Age	Maximum Heart Rate	80% of Maximum Exercise Pulse	75% of Maximum For Heart Disease Patients
20	200	160	150
22	198	158	148
24	196	157	147
26	194	155	145
28	194	154	144
30	190	152	143
32	189	151	142
34	187	150	140
36	186	149	140
38	184	147	138
40	182	146	137
45	179	143	134
50	175	140	131
55	171	137	128
60	160	128	120
65 +	150	120	113

EXERCISE – HOW MUCH IS ENOUGH?

In order to raise your metabolic rate, each exercise session should be at least 12 minutes long at 80 per cent of your ideal pulse rate. It may take you five minutes to get up to this rate, in which case you'll need to exercise for 17 minutes.

If you want to lose weight faster, don't exercise harder, just exercise for longer. As you get fitter you may need to exercise for longer to maintain the 'training' effect. Remember, the more consistently you exercise, even if you're changing from one sport to another, the easier it is to exercise. It's much harder to stop and start.

When you start, especially if you are carrying around a lot of fat, doing 12 minutes of aerobic exercise three times a week will get you fit. Once you are fitter, this level of exercise will maintain your fitness. If you do less, you will lose fitness, and if you exercise six days a week you will get fitter and fitter. It is best to start off exercising three times a week.

THE BLISSS EXERCISE PROGRAMME

The BLISSS Exercise programme is not a set of exercises but a system for checking that what you're doing maximizes your health and metabolic rate.

Base – increase your daily level of basic exercise by walking
Line – more, being energetic and doing things the hard way
I – choose exercises that stimulate you as an individual
S – include exercises that increase your strength
S – include exercises that maintain your suppleness
S – most of all include aerobic exercise for stamina

But remember, you don't have to be fanatical about anything, except not being fanatical!

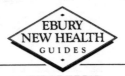

CHAPTER 7

THE METABOLIC DIET

Having explained how and why the Metabolic Diet works, this is where you start losing weight. The Metabolic Diet is the whole approach to slimming because it takes into account all factors that help you increase and balance your metabolic rate. These factors are shown in a nutshell in the diagram below. The next three chapters tell you what you have to do. But first, here are some 'do's and don'ts' which will help you to lose weight faster and feel healthier sooner.

DO'S

Get off to a good start by following the diet and supplements strictly for the first month. In month two the quantity of food increases, and it won't really matter if you bend the rules a little.

Eat as much fruit, vegetables, including sprouts as you can. Half your diet in quantity should be made up from these foods.

Eat all (non-meat) food as raw as possible. All cooking destroys some vitamins and breaks down fibre. Almost all vegetables are tasty raw, and those that need cooking need less than you think. Experiment and see what suits you.

When using oils other than for cooking, for example in mayonnaise or salad dressings, use cold-pressed sunflower, sesame or safflower oils.

Drink at least half a pint of water a day, between meals. For other drinks have diluted fruit juice, herb teas or coffee substitutes.

Keep to the exercise programme. The first two weeks is always the hardest, but after that exercise gets easier and easier.

DON'TS

Avoid sugar and other foods with concentrated sweetness. Honey and maple syrup are only marginally better. Dilute fruit juice and soak dried fruit.

Keep alcohol to a minimum. Certainly drink no more than four glasses of wine, or four pub measures of spirits, or four half pints of beer or lager a week.

Avoid fatty meats like beef, pork and lamb and other high fat foods. Have more vegetarian forms of protein.

Avoid 'processed' and 'fast' foods with long lists of preservatives and additives.

Avoid frying foods. Grill or bake instead. If you do fry use the smallest amount of olive oil or butter for as short a time as possible.

Where possible, avoid foods with added salt, and don't add salt to your food. It isn't needed.

Avoid coffee and cut down on tea consumption. If you are a tea addict, get a smaller pot and cup, make it weaker and have it less often. Drink as much herb tea or coffee substitute as you wish.

Don't stop the diet if you feel worse in the first week. This diet is also a cleansing diet and sometimes the body responds by cleaning out old toxins. This has been known to result in temporary headaches, tiredness, and slight nausea. All this goes away in a couple of days.

STIMULATE YOUR METABOLISM

To stimulate your metabolism and get those pounds dropping off, this diet is best followed as closely as possible for the first 30 days. Each of the 15 daily menu plans is already balanced for health, the prime objective being to give you 300 protein, carbohydrate and fat points. It is also a good chance to find out which recipes suit you best. For Day 16 to Day 30, you can either start again from the beginning or select the menus you liked best.

After the first 30 days you can make up your own metabolic recipes (see Working Out Your Own Metabolic Diet) or adjust these ones to suit your taste. Your target for months 2 and 3 should be 350 protein, carbohydrate and fat points.

STARTING THE METABOLIC DIET

Please note that some recipes are designed for four people, so if you are cooking for less divide the quantities by four or freeze the spare amounts. All fat, carbohydrate and protein points given for each meal are based on the servings for one person.

DAY 1

BREAKFAST
Apple muesli

LUNCH
Cottage cheese and alfalfa sandwich with coleslaw

DINNER
Spicy almond couscous served with watercress salad

SNACKS
One banana, ¼ pint skimmed milk in drinks

Protein Points 280   Carbohydrate Points 320   Fat Points 255

DAY 2

BREAKFAST
Porridge

LUNCH
Potato salad with 1 oz cheese followed by a banana

DINNER
Vegetable casserole, sprinkled with 1 oz Cheddar cheese served on 2 oz brown rice for each person with tomato and beansprout salad, sprinkled with 1 tbsp French dressing

SNACKS
¼ pint skimmed milk with drinks

Protein Points 285   Carbohydrate Points 330   Fat Points 220

DAY 3

BREAKFAST
Pear and cashew yoghurt

LUNCH
Farmhouse vegetable soup (in a thermos if you are working) followed by a tofu sandwich

DINNER
Lentil, courgette and potato casserole served with watercress salad and Vecon potatoes. These are made by adding 3 tbsp Vecon stock to boiled potatoes, once the water has been removed, and continuing to boil for two minutes, coating potatoes with the Vecon stock. A small amount of butter can be added to the potatoes

SNACKS
2 bananas, 1 apple, 1 oz cheese, 1 slice of wholemeal bread and butter and ¼ pint skimmed milk in drinks

Protein Points 280   Carbohydrate Points 280   Fat Points 275

DAY 4

BREAKFAST
Banana yoghurt

LUNCH
Apple and tuna salad and 1 slice wholemeal bread spread very thinly with butter

DINNER
Spaghetti Napolitana served with watercress salad followed by raspberry sorbet

SNACKS
1 banana, 1 orange, 1 apple, 1 oz Cheddar cheese and $\frac{1}{4}$ pint skimmed milk in drinks

Protein Points 305   Carbohydrate Points 320   Fat Points 255

DAY 5

BREAKFAST
Banana yoghurt

LUNCH
Potato salad followed by 4 oz grapes and an apple

DINNER
Farmhouse vegetable soup followed by chicken salad served with a baked potato with 1 oz cottage cheese and $\frac{1}{4}$ oz butter

SNACKS
1 banana and $\frac{1}{4}$ pint skimmed milk in drinks

Protein Points 310   Carbohydrate Points 325   Fat Points 240

DAY 6

——— **BREAKFAST** ———
Porridge

——— **LUNCH** ———
Carrot soup and a tofu sandwich

——— **DINNER** ———
Lentil curry served with 2 oz brown rice per person and rainbow root
salad

——— **SNACKS** ———
1 banana, 1 orange, 1 slice of wholemeal bread and butter and ¼ pint
skimmed milk

Protein Points 305   Carbohydrate Points 340   Fat Points 250

DAY 7

——— **BREAKFAST** ———
Apple muesli

——— **LUNCH** ———
Baked potato (as given in lunch recipes)

——— **DINNER** ———
Mushroom pilaff served with tomato and beansprout salad followed
by baked date and apple

——— **SNACKS** ———
¼ pint skimmed milk

Protein Points 315   Carbohydrate Points 380   Fat Points 95

DAY 8

BREAKFAST
Banana yoghurt

LUNCH
Potato salad with 1 oz Cheddar cheese

DINNER
Lentil soup followed by Tabouli with tomato and beansprout salad

SNACKS
1 orange, 1 apple and $\frac{1}{4}$ pint skimmed milk

Protein Points 270   Carbohydrate Points 315   Fat Points 205

DAY 9

BREAKFAST
Porridge

LUNCH
Cheddar corn salad with 1 piece wholemeal bread and butter

DINNER
Chick-pea feast with spinach and bean salad followed by baked date and apple

SNACKS
1 banana, 1 apple, 6 figs and $\frac{1}{4}$ pint skimmed milk

Protein Points 315   Carbohydrate Points 290   Fat Points 205

DAY 10

BREAKFAST
Pear and cashew yoghurt

LUNCH
Cottage cheese and alfalfa sandwich

DINNER
Vegetable soup followed by baked beans on toast with rainbow root salad and 8 oz Vecon potatoes for each person

SNACKS
2 bananas, 1 apple, 1 piece wholemeal bread and butter and $\frac{1}{4}$ pint skimmed milk

Protein Points 305   Carbohydrate Points 300   Fat Points 175

DAY 11

BREAKFAST
Prune yoghurt

LUNCH
Cottage cheese and alfalfa sandwich and coleslaw

DINNER
Stuffed potatoes with rainbow root salad followed by apricot whisk

SNACKS
1 banana, 2 apples and $\frac{1}{4}$ pint skimmed milk

Protein Points 295   Carbohydrate Points 355   Fat Points 195

DAY 12

BREAKFAST
Banana yoghurt

LUNCH
Apple tuna salad followed by an apple

DINNER
Hummus followed by chestnut hot pot with spinach and bean salad, followed by fruit salad

SNACKS
¼ pint skimmed milk

Protein Points 315   Carbohydrate Points 310   Fat Points 200

DAY 13

BREAKFAST
Fruit milk shake

LUNCH
Lentil soup and coleslaw

DINNER
Courgette Quickie served on a bed of rice (2 oz per person) with watercress salad, followed by apricot whisk

SNACKS
1 banana, 1 apple and ¼ pint skimmed milk

Protein Points 305   Carbohydrate Points 320   Fat Points 230

DAY 14

BREAKFAST
Apple muesli

LUNCH
Potato salad

DINNER
Fish pie with watercress salad

SNACKS
1 banana, 1 orange and ¼ pint skimmed milk

Protein Points 305   Carbohydrate Points 290   Fat Points 155

DAY 15

BREAKFAST
Fruit cocktail

LUNCH
Hummus and Cheddar corn salad

DINNER
Kedgeree followed by fruit salad

SNACKS
1 banana, 4 oz grapes, 3 figs, 10 almonds and ¼ pint milk

Protein Points 290   Carbohydrate Points 300   Fat Points 250

SHOPPING LIST

Some of the foods used in these recipes may be new to you. All of them are readily available in either your local health food shop or good greengrocer's. Everything you need to buy for the first 15 days is on this list, together with our favourite recommended brands.

Shopping List	Recommended Brands
Skimmed milk	fresh from your milkman
Very low fat natural yoghurt	Loseley
Lots of fresh vegetables	
Garlic	
Lots of fresh fruit – particularly bananas	
Dried fruit – apricots, dates, raisins	
Nuts – almonds, cashews, coconut	
Wheatgerm – not stabilized	Jordans
Natural vanilla essence	Ethos or Lane's
Rolled oats	
Honey	
Mayonnaise	
Cottage cheese	
Tofu	
Tahini	Harmony
Shoyu	Sunwheel or Harmony
Alfalfa seeds or sprouts	
Lentils – brown and green	
Chick-peas	
Red kidney beans	
Brown rice	
Couscous	
Bulghar	
Dried chestnuts	
Baked beans	Whole Earth
Wholemeal spaghetti	
Olive oil – cold pressed	
Vecon, vegetable stock	Vecon
Vegetable stock cubes	Hugli or Morga
Bouillon powder	Hugli or Morga
Yeast extract – low salt	Natex
Cider vinegar	Aspall
Wholemeal flour	
Sugar-free de luxe muesli	
Quark or low fat soft cheese	
Herbs – mixed, cumin, thyme, basil	
Herb teas	Celestial Seasonings
Dandelion coffee	Symingtons
Barleycup	Barleycup

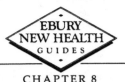

CHAPTER 8

METABOLIC
SUPPLEMENTS

WHILE diet is definitely the place to start, diet alone cannot supply the optimal levels of vital vitamins and minerals to maximize your metabolism. A crucial part of the Metabolic Diet is a special daily programme of vitamin and mineral supplements.

The Metabolic Diet also includes daily supplements of Glucomannan fibre. This remarkable fibre, explained fully in Chapter 5, has been shown to cause weight loss of between seven and 14 lb over three months, without any change to diet or exercise.

THIS IS YOUR IDEAL DAILY PROGRAMME:

Supplement	With Breakfast	Before Lunch	Before Dinner	With Dinner
Vitamin C 1,000 mg	1			1
Multivitamin	1			
B Complex	1			
B6 100 mg + Zinc 10 mg				1
B3 100 mg + Chromium 100 mcg	1			
Glucomannan Fibre 500 mg		3	3	

HOW AND WHEN TO TAKE THEM

All vitamins and minerals are best taken within 15 minutes of a meal. Before, after or during makes no difference. Taking them twice a day maximizes their effect, but if you're particularly forgetful, taking them once a day in the morning is far better than forgetting to take them two days out of seven.

Glucomannan is best taken 30 minutes before a major meal. Some people recommend taking one in the morning, two before lunch and three before dinner. If lunch, tea-time and dinner are the times you would be most likely to over-eat then you may prefer to take three before lunch and three before dinner. Always take Glucomannan with a very large glass of water.

One in 20 people experience slight flatulence and even constipation during the first three days. This soon subsides and occurs simply because the body has not been used to large quantities of fibre.

HOW LONG SHOULD I TAKE SUPPLEMENTS?

Glucomannan is only needed for the first three months. The other supplements can be taken indefinitely. However, once you have reached your target weight, I recommend you stop taking the vitamin B6 + Zinc and the B3 + Chromium, and replace these with a good Multi Mineral tablet. This should provide a basic level of zinc and chromium, while the B3 and B6 is already contained in the Multivite and B Complex in sufficient quantity for on-going use.

WHICH SUPPLEMENTS SHOULD I BUY?

There are many good makes of supplements, and some of my favourites are Health+Plus, Healthcrafts, Quest, Meadowcroft and Cantassium. But the important thing is to check that the dosage given matches the doses shown in Chapter 3. Many people try to buy the cheapest Multivite only to find they are paying half the price for a tenth of the dose. After all, you wouldn't expect a headache to go away with a tenth of an aspirin. Most health shop assistants can advise you on the best combination of supplements to meet your needs.

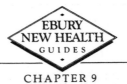
CHAPTER 9

MONITORING YOUR FITNESS AND FATLESSNESS

Most people start diets hoping to lose in a month what they gained in a year. They vow to never eat chocolate again and to exercise every day. This approach usually ends in failure.

My advice to you, having worked with hundreds of overweight people, is to take it one step at a time. Set yourself targets for changing your diet and taking exercise that you know you will achieve. The weight will look after itself. It is far better to gradually change your lifestyle, than to take four steps forward and then three steps back, by following an over-ambitious regime.

After all, we often eat because we are under pressure or stressed. Boredom, frustration, anger, lack of direction all lead to feelings that can be temporarily suppressed with food. Even making small dietary changes is, in the first instance, stressful. It takes time to adjust. So don't add to your stress by expecting too much from yourself, and then failing to meet your targets. You took years to get fat. Does it really matter if you take months, rather than weeks, to lose it?

MONITORING YOUR WEIGHT

Don't forget the percentage of your weight that is fat is a far more important statistic than your weight. So don't rely on your scales as the only means of checking your progress. As you begin to convert some of that fat to muscle through exercise, you won't lose much weight, since muscle is heavier than fat, but you will lose inches, since muscle is more compact than fat. Muscle cells are metabolically active and therefore have the capacity to burn off fat, while fat cells don't. So first you've got to make the muscle, then lose the weight.

The chart below shows you your ideal weight for height. These figures are calculated from life insurance figures. If you're within the ideal range, don't lose more than 4 lb a month. If you are above the ideal range don't target to lose more than 6 lb a month.

YOUR IDEAL WEIGHT
(Weight in pounds, wearing indoor clothing)

Men of ages 25 and over		Women of ages 25 and over	
Height	Weight	Height	Weight
5' 1"	112–129	4' 8"	92–107
5' 2"	115–133	4' 9"	94–110
5' 3"	118–136	4' 10"	96–113
5' 4"	121–139	4' 11"	99–116
5' 5"	124–143	5' 0"	102–119
5' 6"	128–147	5' 1"	105–122
5' 7"	132–152	5' 2"	108–126
5' 8"	136–156	5' 3"	111–130
5' 9"	140–160	5' 4"	114–135
5' 10"	144–165	5' 5"	118–139
5' 11"	148–170	5' 6"	122–143
6' 0"	152–175	5' 7"	126–147
6' 1"	156–180	5' 8"	130–151
6' 2"	160–185	5' 9"	134–155
6' 3"	164–190	5' 10"	138–159

MONITORING YOUR EXERCISE

There are many different forms of exercise, all with different advantages and disadvantages. To find out which suit you best read Chapter 4. Once you've selected your preferred exercise or exercises, since variety is the spice of life, the following chart will help you to make sure you're doing enough to raise your metabolic rate.

Since different forms of exercise have differing degrees of 'aerobic hardness' this chart shows you how long you need to do each exercise to raise your metabolic rate. Whatever the exercise, a 'unit' of exercise represents the same metabolic effect. Fifteen units of exercise a week will raise your metabolic rate. Set your weekly target at 15 units, and your 'reward target' at 20 units. When you hit 20 units reward yourself by doing something you really enjoy. Go dancing, see a film, buy yourself some nice clothes, or go out to dinner – but don't eat too much!

EXERCISE TIMES FOR FITNESS

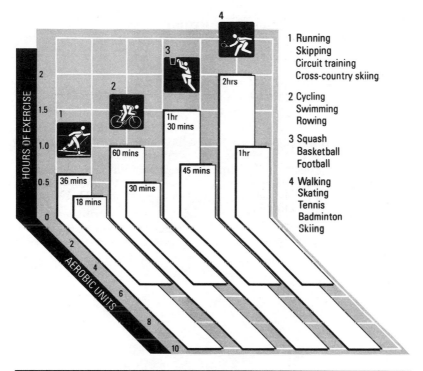

1 Running
  Skipping
  Circuit training
  Cross-country skiing

2 Cycling
  Swimming
  Rowing

3 Squash
  Basketball
  Football

4 Walking
  Skating
  Tennis
  Badminton
  Skiing

MONITORING YOUR DIET

With the Batterham Diet Balancer monitoring your diet is easy. For the first month your target is to eat 300 protein, 300 carbohydrate and 300 fat points each day. You'll find it's never that accurate. The important thing is to keep fat points below 300 units, and carbohydrate points at or above 300 points. When you've completed the first month successfully reward yourself with something really special.

For month two and onwards, it gets easy. Just keep your fat points below 350, and aim for 350 protein points and 350 or more carbohydrate points. You will lose weight on this diet, although it will feel like you're eating masses.

Once you've reached your ideal weight, this can be maintained on 400 protein, carbohydrate and fat points. In fact, by this stage you certainly won't need to work out the points for everything you eat. You'll just know what's right for you. You can keep a record of your points on the Health and Fitness Diary pages at the end of this chapter.

MONITORING YOUR ENERGY

Monitoring your energy allows you to see how much your energy improves during the first three months. It takes approximately 30 seconds once a week. This is what you have to do.

A score of 100 per cent means that your energy level is the most you could imagine, and 0 per cent represents the worst you could possibly imagine.

What is the lowest energy score you have ever experienced? Now, how would you rate your average level of energy during the last week? Log this on your graph by shading in the WEEK ONE area up to the percentage score for the last week. The score for WEEK TWO represents your first week on the Metabolic Diet.

Pick a time, preferably right now, when you can routinely monitor your rating for energy. As this will be your own subjective rating, the actual scores do not matter – it is the relative change over the next three months which is important. So don't be over-concerned about where you place your first score just as long as you leave room for improvement.

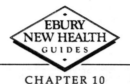

CHAPTER 10

METABOLIC RECIPES

Some people equate healthy eating and 'health' foods with eating endless salad, 'soya' sausages and beansprouts! You'll find these recipes a pleasant surprise.

All recipes are sugar-free, using the natural sweetness present in fruits. They are also low in salt. If you're used to eating salt, this diet, together with the supplements, will improve your sense of taste. They are also high in fibre, so you don't need to add bran. We've also selected foods that are packed with vitamin vitality.

But most of all, each recipe is balanced to promote optimum metabolism. The protein, carbohydrate and fat points are given for each dish. If you choose a higher fat breakfast, have a lower fat lunch. The objective is to end up with approximately equal scores for protein, carbohydrate and fat.

BREAKFASTS

APPLE MUESLI

Buy a good quality deluxe, sugar-free muesli from your local health food shop; this will have more nuts and fruits than average.

YOU WILL NEED
2 oz (50 g) muesli deluxe
200 ml (8 fl oz) skimmed
    milk
1 apple

1 Soak muesli overnight in $\frac{1}{4}$ pint water.
2 Add milk and grated apple.

PROTEIN 70   CARBO 95   FAT 40
SERVES ONE

PEAR AND CASHEW YOGHURT

Low fat, live yoghurt is a first class food, unlike its commercial counterpart, in which most bacteria have been destroyed for a longer shelf life. Live yoghurt is packed with good bacteria that have a spring-cleaning effect on your digestive system, as well as being a fine source of protein. Jazzed up with pear and cashew, it's a great way to start the day.

YOU WILL NEED
1 pear
5 oz (125 g) very low fat
   yoghurt
A handful of cashews
1 tbsp wheatgerm

1 Chop pear and combine with all other ingredients.

PROTEIN 125   CARBO 45   FAT 95
SERVES ONE

BANANA BREAKFAST

Banana and crunchy coconut chips are the best foods to add to yoghurt, because the citric acid in fruits like oranges rapidly destroys the beneficial bacteria.

YOU WILL NEED
1 banana
5 oz (125 g) very low fat
   yoghurt
1 tbsp of toasted coconut
   chips
5 dates

1 Chop banana and combine with all the remaining ingredients.

PROTEIN 40   CARBO 65   FAT 35
SERVES ONE

FRUIT COCKTAIL

Use whatever fruits are in season – grated apple and banana, orange and banana, orange and peach or a mix of strawberries, raspberries, red- and blackcurrants.

YOU WILL NEED
1½ tbsp desiccated coconut
¼ tsp vanilla essence
4 oz (100 g) fruit

1 Liquidize all ingredients together with some ice.

PROTEIN 15   CARBO 30   FAT 80
SERVES ONE

FRUIT MILKSHAKE

This is really a hundred different breakfasts depending on the fruit you use. Try it with peaches, and strawberries, or banana and fresh dates. As a treat have a mango milkshake.

YOU WILL NEED
2 oz (50 g) fruit
1 tbsp ground almonds
1 lbsp desiccated coconut
¼ pint (150 ml) skimmed milk

1 Liquidize fruit, almonds, coconut and some ice.
2 Add milk and liquidize again.

PROTEIN 40   CARBO 35   FAT 100
SERVES ONE

SCOTS PORRIDGE

On a cold winter day, nothing can be more warming than porridge. Oats contain special factors that are known to promote a healthy heart and arteries and are full of fibre and complex carbohydrates.

YOU WILL NEED
½ pint (300 ml) water
½ pint (300 ml) skimmed milk
1 oz (25 g) porridge oats
1 tsp honey

1 Put the water and half the milk in a saucepan and sprinkle in the oats.
2 Bring to the boil and boil for five minutes, stirring all the time.
3 Serve with milk and a little honey.

PROTEIN 70   CARBO 85   FAT 15
SERVES ONE

PRUNE AND ALMOND YOGHURT

The secret to prunes is soaking them. All dried fruits taste far better soaked overnight. They are more filling and are better for you, being less concentrated in simple sugar. Try this breakfast and you'll see.

YOU WILL NEED
4 oz (100 g) prunes
5 oz (125 g) very low fat yoghurt
½ oz (15 g) almonds

1 Soak prunes in water overnight.
2 Remove stones.
3 Liquidize with yoghurt.
4 Serve sprinkled with chopped almonds.

PROTEIN 50   CARBO 85   FAT 45
SERVES ONE

EASY PACKED LUNCHES

CARROT COLESLAW

Cabbages are packed with vitamins and minerals. So are carrots, high in vitamin A, and onions, high in sulphur containing amino acids, which help to remove toxins from the body.

YOU WILL NEED
1 lb (450 g) white or red
  cabbage
8 oz (225 g) carrots
4 oz (100 g) onion
4 oz (100 g) raisins
2 tbsp mayonnaise
2 tbsp very low fat yoghurt
1 tbsp skimmed milk

1 Finely chop cabbage, carrots and onion.
2 Mix all ingredients.
3 Eat with celery and carrot sticks.

PROTEIN 20   CARBO 40   FAT 40
SERVES FOUR

POTATO SALAD

YOU WILL NEED
2 lb (900 g) cold boiled
  potatoes
8 blades fresh chives (or
  dried)
2 tbsp mayonnaise
2 tbsp yoghurt
1 tbsp skimmed milk

1 Dice potatoes.
2 Add chives and remaining ingredients.

PROTEIN 27   CARBO 63   FAT 42
SERVES FOUR

BAKED POTATO

Potatoes are always left out of slimming recipes, but they are one of the few foods you could live off entirely. But do eat the skins since they're full of fibre. When making your own baked potatoes cook them for as short a time as possible, till they are cooked but crispy inside. Over-cooking turns potato's complex carbohydrate into simple sugar.

YOU WILL NEED
For the filling
5 oz (150 g) cottage cheese
10 slices cucumber
4 blades chives

1 Buy a ready cooked baked potato at a takeaway shop (without butter) and add a home-made filling of cottage cheese, chives and cucumber.

PROTEIN 130   CARBO 95   FAT 5
SERVES ONE

TOFU AND ALFALFA SANDWICH

Tofu is a curd made from soya beans. It's the staple food of half of China and is an excellent low fat source of protein. Alfalfa sprouts contain saponins which help lower cholesterol levels. Together, they make a delicious sandwich filler.

YOU WILL NEED
5 oz (150 g) tofu
1 tsp tahini
1 tsp shoyu
8 slices wholemeal bread
  spread very thinly with
  butter
5 oz (150 g) alfalfa sprouts

1 Mix all filling ingredients thoroughly.
2 Fill sandwiches (this will make four rounds) with tofu filling and plenty of alfalfa sprouts (or cress).

PROTEIN 35   CARBO 30   FAT 55
SERVES FOUR, filling will keep in fridge for many days

COTTAGE CHEESE AND ALFALFA SANDWICH

Cottage cheese is the lowest fat cheese and contains the minerals high in all milk products. Combined with alfalfa sprouts, it makes a great sandwich mix.

YOU WILL NEED FOR EACH
SANDWICH
2 oz (50 g) cottage cheese
large handful alfalfa sprouts
2 slices lightly buttered
   wholemeal bread

PROTEIN 70   CARBO 30   FAT 40
SERVES ONE

STARTERS

OREGANO LENTIL SOUP

Lentils are excellent carbohydrate rich foods, which have a minimal effect on raising blood sugar level and provide good protein as well as plenty of vitamins and minerals. This is an excellent winter dish that only takes 25 minutes.

YOU WILL NEED
8 oz (225 g) brown or
   continental lentils –
   washed
1¼ pints (750 ml) water
14 oz (400 g) tin tomatoes
   (or 1 lb (450 g) fresh
   tomatoes)
2 tsp oregano
2 cloves garlic, crushed
1 tsp Vecon
freshly ground black pepper

1 Simmer lentils until tender in water in a covered pan.
2 Add tomatoes, oregano, garlic, Vecon and pepper.
3 Simmer for a further five minutes.
4 Add pepper to taste.

PROTEIN 70   CARBO 45   FAT 5
SERVES FOUR, Cooking Time
1 hour 5 minutes

FARMHOUSE VEGETABLE SOUP

There are as many different kinds of vegetable soup as there are vegetables. Try leek and potato, or cauliflower, or carrot or a combination of swede, carrot, turnip and parsnip.

YOU WILL NEED
*1¹/₂ lb (700 g) chopped fresh
vegetables, e.g. carrots,
celery, leeks, potatoes,
courgettes, tomatoes,
cauliflower*
1 medium onion
*1 low-salt vegetable stock
cube*
2 tsp mixed herbs

1 Slice the onion and simmer it in a little water until it is soft.
2 Add the chopped vegetables (a combination of those suggested or one single one can be used).
3 Add herbs and the stock cube.
4 Cover with water and simmer until all the vegetables are just soft.
5 Liquidize or purée and serve the soup hot.

PROTEIN 8   CARBO 16   FAT 0
*SERVES FOUR, Cooking Time
30 minutes*

CARROT SOUP IN THE RAW

Ever had a hot, raw soup? This soup is made cold and heated gently, keeping all the vitamin and mineral content intact. It's also full of fibre. Don't overheat it.

YOU WILL NEED
1 lb (450 g) carrots
4 oz (100 g) ground almonds
*¹/₂ pint (300 ml) skimmed
milk*
1 vegetable stock cube
*1 tsp mixed herbs (fresh if
possible)*

1 Chop the carrots and place in food processor and process until a fine purée is achieved.
2 Add other ingredients and process until mixed.
3 Warm very gently in a pan.

PROTEIN 40   CARBO 20   FAT 90
SERVES FOUR

HUMMUS

Chick-peas, also known as garbanzo beans, have a unique taste which combines well with tahini, a paste made from sesame seeds. Chick-peas can also be sprouted first, increasing their vitamin content.

YOU WILL NEED
4 oz (100 g) chick-peas
1 garlic clove, crushed
1 tbsp olive oil
juice of 1 lemon
2 tbsp natural yoghurt
1 tbsp tahini (available from
   health food shops)
freshly ground black pepper
8 slices wholemeal or 8
   oatcakes (these will have a
   higher fat level than
   bread)

1 Soak the chick-peas overnight, cover with fresh water and simmer for 45 minutes with the garlic.
2 Put chick-peas, garlic, lemon juice, tahini, yoghurt, olive oil in a liquidizer and purée adding extra water if necessary.
3 Add freshly ground black pepper to taste.
4 Serve on oatcakes or toast (no butter needed).

PROTEIN 70   CARBO 55   FAT 55
SERVES FOUR, Cooking Time
45 minutes
Suitable for freezing

TOMATO AND HORSERADISH SALAD

A nice side-salad for a main meal. Select good and tasty tomatoes, as this makes all the difference.

YOU WILL NEED
4 large tomatoes
FOR DRESSING
4 oz (100 g) Quark or low
   fat soft cheese
2 tbsp skimmed milk
3 tsp horseradish sauce
2 tbsp lemon juice
2 tbsp fresh, chopped parsley
   or chives
4 slices wholemeal bread

1 Mix all ingredients for dressing thoroughly.
2 Slice tomatoes and arrange on individual plates.
3 Top with dressing.
4 Serve with wholemeal bread – no butter.

PROTEIN 40   CARBO 20   FAT 20
SERVES FOUR

CALIFORNIAN GOLD

More of a main course than a starter. This dish is excellent for unleashing your artistic talent.

YOU WILL NEED
1 apple
1 banana
1 nectarine
1 kiwi fruit
8 grapes (deseeded)
lemon juice
6 oz (175 g) cottage cheese
alfalfa sprouts

1 Slice fruit and arrange on individual dishes.
2 Sprinkle with lemon juice and top with cottage cheese and alfalfa sprouts.

PROTEIN 35   CARBO 25   FAT 5
SERVES FOUR

SALADS

RAINBOW ROOT SALAD

This colourful combination of carrots, parsnips and beetroots is more filling than you think. Go easy on the beetroot and parsnips as their strong tastes can overpower the carrots.

YOU WILL NEED
3 medium carrots, grated
1 small parsnip, grated
1 medium beetroot, grated
parsley, finely chopped

1 Combine three root vegetables.
2 Mix with island dressing (see page 85). Garnish with parsley.
3 To make dressing, liquidize carrot and tomato, add in rest of ingredients including nutmeg to taste and mix thoroughly.

ISLAND DRESSING

1 small carrot
1 small tomato
1 tbsp tofu
1 tsp mayonnaise
1 tsp ground almonds
$^1/_2$ tsp Vecon
1 tbsp skimmed milk
nutmeg, grated

PROTEIN 5 CARBO 5 FAT 10
SERVES FOUR

SPINACH AND BEAN SALAD

Spinach is an underestimated salad food, but care must be taken in preparing spinach leaves.

YOU WILL NEED
1 lb (450 g) fresh spinach
3 tbsp minced onion
14 oz (350 g) cooked and
  cooled red or black kidney
  beans (available ready
  cooked in tins)

FOR THE DRESSING
$^1/_2$ tbsp olive oil
$1^1/_2$ tbsp lemon juice
$^1/_2$ tsp bouillion powder

PROTEIN 55 CARBO 25 FAT 20
SERVES FOUR

1 Carefully strip the spinach leaves from the stalk and soak them in a tub of cold water.
2 Lift leaves and rinse under running water.
3 Drain and pat dry.
4 Chop the leaves coarsely and chop the stems into small pieces.
5 Put the spinach in a large bowl and toss with the onions and half the beans.
6 Arrange the rest of the beans on top.
7 Mix the dressing ingredients together well.
8 Sprinkle the dressing over the salad.

WATERCRESS SALAD

Watercress makes a good change from lettuce. Use half watercress and half lettuce.

YOU WILL NEED
For the salad
1/2 bunch watercress
1/3 iceberg lettuce, sliced
20 or so slices cucumber
1 green pepper
3 handfuls alfalfa sprouts

FOR THE FRENCH DRESSING
4 tbsp olive oil
2 tbsp cider vinegar
1 tsp French mustard
1 tsp mixed herbs
1/4 tsp honey
clove of garlic, crushed

PROTEIN 0   CARBO 5   FAT 15
SERVES FOUR

1 Combine all salad ingredients.
2 To make French dressing, put all ingredients in a screw-top jar and shake vigorously. The quantities given will make enough for many salads, so keep it in the fridge and use as required.
3 Toss with 1 tbsp French dressing.

CHEDDAR CORN SALAD WITH CASHEW DRESSING

A fresh corn picked at the right time tastes so sweet you can eat it like a fruit. As the corn ages, the sugar form changes and five minutes cooking is needed to bring out the taste.

YOU WILL NEED
For the salad
2 oz (50 g) Cheddar cheese,
grated
1/2 iceberg lettuce, chopped
1 small green pepper, sliced
2 handfuls alfalfa sprouts
kernels cut from 2 corn-
on-the-cobs or 8 oz
(200 g) frozen corn cooked
very slightly
4 oz (100 g) cherry tomato
halves to garnish

FOR THE DRESSING
1 tbsp ground cashews
1 tbsp natural yoghurt
1 tsp mayonnaise
1 tsp skimmed milk

PROTEIN 20   CARBO 15   FAT 15
SERVES FOUR

1 Combine all salad ingredients.
2 Mix the dressing ingredients in a bowl.
3 Toss the salad in the dressing.

TOMATO AND BEANSPROUT SALAD

YOU WILL NEED
4 large tomatoes
beansprouts
1 tbsp French dressing as
opposite

PROTEIN 20   CARBO 10   FAT 15
SERVES FOUR

1 Slice tomatoes and mix with beansprouts and dressing.

MAIN MEALS

VEGETABLE CASSEROLE

There are many variations to this basic theme. Although it takes a while to cook, the preparation takes only 15 minutes.

YOU WILL NEED
1 tbsp olive oil
2 large onions, sliced
1 lb (450 g) carrots, sliced
1 lb (450 g) potatoes, cut
  into bite sized pieces
1 medium cauliflower,
  broken into florets
8 oz (250 g) mushrooms,
  wiped and sliced
2 tbsp wholemeal flour
1 pint (600 ml) water
2 vegetable stock cubes
1 tbsp tomato purée
2 bay leaves
black pepper

1 Heat the oil in a large saucepan and fry the onions for five minutes.
2 Add the rest of the vegetables and fry for four minutes, stirring often.
3 Sprinkle in the flour.
4 Add water, stock cubes, tomato purée, bay leaves and pepper, and bring to the boil.
5 Transfer to a heatproof casserole and bake for 1 hour at 190°C (375°F) gas mark 5.
6 Remove bay leaves before serving.

PROTEIN 40   CARBO 50   FAT 25
SERVES FOUR, Cooking Time 1 hour

COURGETTE QUICKIE

Courgettes have a very special taste which is brought out to the full in this recipe. It's great served with rice or wholewheat spaghetti, or just on its own.

YOU WILL NEED
1 oz (25 g) butter
1 large onion
1 lb (450 g) courgettes,
  thinly sliced
4 large tomatoes, sliced
3 cloves garlic, crushed
freshly ground black pepper
2 oz (50 g) Cheddar cheese,
  finely grated
4 tbsp fresh breadcrumbs
PROTEIN 40   CARBO 25   FAT 65
SERVES FOUR, Cooking Time
15 minutes

1 Melt the butter in a frying pan.
2 Fry the onion until lightly coloured.
3 Add courgettes, tomatoes and garlic, cover and simmer, stirring occasionally, for about 15 minutes or until tender but still crisp.
4 Season with freshly ground black pepper.
5 Pour into a flameproof dish and sprinkle with cheese and breadcrumbs and brown quickly under a hot grill.

FISH PIE

This is my favourite fish recipe. Make sure you ask for colouring-free smoked haddock. Smoked haddock was never bright yellow and the dyes used are not good for you anyway.

YOU WILL NEED
13 oz (325 g) combined white
  fish and colouring-free
  smoked haddock
½ oz (10 g) butter
1 tbsp wholemeal flour
5 fl oz (150 ml) skimmed
  milk
5 oz (150 g) prawns
4 oz (100 g) mushrooms
2 tsp mixed herbs
freshly ground black pepper
1½ lb (700 g) potatoes
2–3 tbsp skimmed milk
2 oz (50 g) Cheddar cheese
PROTEIN 175   CARBO 55   FAT 55
SERVES FOUR, Cooking Time
30 minutes, suitable for freezing

1 Steam fish above small amount of water for 15 minutes.
2 Meanwhile, make a béchamel sauce out of the butter, flour and milk.
3 Combine fish, sauce, prawns, mushrooms, herbs and pepper.
4 Boil the potatoes and mash with the milk. Season with freshly ground black pepper.
5 Place in oven-proof dish and top with the mashed potatoes.
6 Sprinkle with grated cheese and bake for 30 minutes at 200°C (400°F) gas mark 6.

KEDGEREE

When cooking brown rice it is important not to overcook it. Apart from the fact that it will be stodgy and unpleasant, overcooking it transforms it from a complex to a simple carbohydrate. The rice should still be in separate grains and not have the appearance of splitting out of its skin.

YOU WILL NEED
*12 oz (300 g) colouring-free
  smoked haddock*
8 oz (200 g) brown rice
1¼ (750 ml) pints water
1 egg
parsley
paprika

PROTEIN 120   CARBO 70   FAT 50
*SERVES FOUR, Cooking Time
25 minutes*

1 Bring water to the boil, add rice and boil for 25 minutes with lid tightly on.
2 Meanwhile steam the haddock in a little water.
3 Combine the flaked haddock, butter and rice.
4 Arrange on a dish and decorate with hard-boiled egg slices, fresh chopped parsley and paprika.

SPAGHETTI NAPOLITANA

If you've never tried wholewheat spaghetti or buckwheat spaghetti this is the recipe to try them with. I prefer buckwheat spaghetti but you have to be a bit careful how you cook it. Bring it to the boil, then add cold water, then bring it to the boil. Do this twice for best results.

YOU WILL NEED
*12 oz (300 g) wholemeal
  spaghetti*
2 medium onions
2 tbsp olive oil
3 medium carrots
8 oz (225 g) mushrooms
1 clove garlic
1 small green pepper
4 oz (100 g) tomato purée
*2 tsp Vecon or vegetable
  stock*
2 tsp thyme

PROTEIN 85   CARBO 115   FAT 45
*SERVES FOUR, Cooking Time
20 minutes
Suitable for freezing (sauce only)*

1 Heat oil in a large saucepan.
2 Add sliced onion, then add crushed garlic, carrots, green pepper and mushrooms.
3 Sauté for five minutes.
4 Add Vecon, thyme and tomato purée.
5 Add water to easily cover and simmer for 20 minutes.
6 Process briefly in a food processor or liquidizer.
7 Meanwhile, put spaghetti in plenty of boiling water and boil for 12 minutes. Drain.
8 Serve the spaghetti topped with the sauce.

CHICKEN SALAD

YOU WILL NEED
cold meat from ¹/₂ a small
4 lb (1.8 kg) roast chicken
3 Cox's apples, cored and
chopped into cubes
3 sticks of celery, chopped
10 oz (275 g) cold boiled
potatoes cut into cubes
5 tbsp (75 ml) pint
mayonnaise
2 tsp horseradish sauce
5 tbsp (75 ml) pint skimmed
milk
¹/₃ iceberg lettuce
red pepper, to garnish

1 Combine all ingredients, except the pepper and lettuce, and pile on a large plate.
2 Decorate with the iceberg lettuce round the edges and three rings of red pepper on top.

PROTEIN 160 CARBO 35 FAT 90
SERVES FOUR

SPICY ALMOND COUSCOUS

This is a variation on a Moroccan dish. The main ingredient is couscous which is an excellent complex carbohydrate food.

YOU WILL NEED
1 tbsp olive oil
8 oz (225 g) courgettes, sliced
1 medium onion, sliced
8 oz (225 g) mushrooms,
sliced
2 oz (50 g) raisins
2 oz (50 g) flaked almonds
14 oz (400 g) tin tomatoes
(or fresh ones)
1 medium red pepper,
chopped
2 medium carrots, sliced
1 tsp pepper or chilli sauce
(or ¹/₂ tsp chilli powder)
8 oz (225 g) couscous
1¹/₂ pints (900 ml) boiling
water

1 Heat oil in a large saucepan.
2 Add the onion and sauté for two minutes.
3 Add rest of the vegetables and sauté for a further two minutes.
4 Add tomatoes, pepper sauce, almonds, raisins and enough water to cover.
5 Simmer until vegetables are not quite soft – about 20 minutes.
6 Meanwhile pour boiling water over couscous and leave to stand for 15 minutes, serve vegetables on a bed of couscous.

PROTEIN 75 CARBO 100 FAT 70
SERVES FOUR, Cooking Time 20 minutes

LENTIL CURRY

Lentil curry is good on its own or served with brown rice.

YOU WILL NEED
1 medium onion, chopped
8 oz (225 g) red lentils
1 tbsp olive oil
1–2 tsp curry powder
1 pint (500 ml) water
1 tsp yeast extract
1 tbsp tomato purée
2 hard-boiled eggs, sliced

PROTEIN 100   CARBO 55   FAT 55
SERVES FOUR, Cooking Time 1 hour
5 minutes

1 Heat the oil gently in a pan and fry the onion in it for five minutes.
2 Add lentils, curry powder, water, yeast extract and tomato purée.
3 Bring to boil and simmer over low heat until lentils are soft and liquid is absorbed. Add more water if needed.
4 Turn into serving dish. Garnish with sliced eggs.

STUFFED PEPPERS

YOU WILL NEED
4 medium peppers
1 medium onion
1 clove garlic, crushed
1 oz (25 g) butter
4 oz (100 g) mushrooms, wiped and chopped
1/2 pint (300 ml) hot water (not from the hot tap)
1 tsp yeast extract
1 egg, beaten
1 tbsp chopped parsley
8 oz (225 g) tomatoes, sliced
brown rice
black pepper

PROTEIN 25   CARBO 15   FAT 50
SERVES FOUR, Cooking Time
30 minutes
Suitable for freezing

1 Cook peppers in boiling water for five minutes. Cut off tops and scrape out seeds with a spoon.
2 Melt butter in frying pan and gently fry onion, garlic and tomatoes until softened.
3 Add rice, mushrooms, water and yeast extract. Simmer until liquid is absorbed and rice cooked, add more hot water if needed.
4 Add egg, parsley and black pepper.
5 Cool a little. Stuff the peppers and place on an oiled, shallow ovenproof dish, and place tops back on.
6 Brush peppers lightly with oil.
7 Bake on top shelf of oven at 200°C (400°F) gas mark 6 for about 30 minutes.

MUSHROOM AND RAISIN PILAFF

Mushrooms can be eaten raw in salads, or cooked as in this delicious pilaff. The secret is to cook them slowly. Adding a little water helps bring out their juices.

YOU WILL NEED
8 oz (225 g) brown rice
1/2 oz (15 g) butter
1 tbsp olive oil
1 large onion, chopped
1 pint (600 ml) hot water
2 oz (50 g) raisins
8 oz (225 g) frozen peas
8 oz (225 g) mushrooms, sliced
1 tsp yeast extract
1 tsp finely chopped root ginger
2 tbsp chopped parsley

PROTEIN 50 CARBO 100 FAT 50
SERVES FOUR, Cooking Time
40 minutes

1 Gently heat the oil and butter in a heavy frying pan and fry the rice in it until pale brown. Add onion and cook for a further five minutes.
2 Add water, raisins and mushrooms, cover and simmer until liquid is absorbed and rice just tender. Add more hot water if needed.
3 Stir in yeast extract and ginger.
4 Cook frozen peas, drain and add to rice mixture.
5 Serve garnished with parsley.

TABOULI

Tabouli is a traditional vegetarian dish using bulgar, which is cracked wheat. It's an excellent source of complex carbohydrate.

YOU WILL NEED
8 oz (225 g) bulgar (cracked wheat)
1 onion, finely chopped
1 bunch finely chopped parsley
3 tbsp fresh mint
3 tbsp olive oil
6 tbsp lemon juice
1/4 cucumber, diced small
freshly ground black pepper
lettuce leaves, to serve

PROTEIN 45 CARBO 70 FAT 65
SERVES FOUR

1 Soak bulgar for 1–2 hours in cold water.
2 Drain bulgar.
3 Mix other ingredients – add more lemon if necessary.
4 Serve on lettuce leaves in a bowl.

TUNA AND CHICK-PEA FEAST

YOU WILL NEED
6 oz (175 g) chick-peas
3 hard-boiled eggs, chopped
7 oz (200 g) tuna in brine,
    drained and flaked
1 small onion, finely chopped
1 tbsp cider vinegar
2 tbsp olive oil
3 tbsp parsley, chopped
1 tbsp chives, chopped
$^1/_2$ tsp mustard
black pepper

PROTEIN 140   CARBO 30   FAT 130
SERVES FOUR, Cooking Time
45 minutes

1 Soak chick-peas overnight and then boil for 45 minutes in plenty of water.
2 Mix chick-peas with eggs, flaked tuna and onion.
3 Mix the rest of the ingredients in a screw top jar, shaking vigorously.
4 Pour over chick-pea mixture and serve on a large dish.

LENTIL, COURGETTE AND POTATO HOTPOT

YOU WILL NEED
8 oz (225 g) green lentils
2 pints (1.2 litres) water
3 bay leaves
1 onion
1 tbsp olive oil
12 oz (350 g) courgettes
2 cloves garlic, crushed
juice of $^1/_2$ lemon
basil
$^1/_2$ tsp ground cumin
8 oz (225 g) potatoes
black pepper

PROTEIN 20   CARBO 20   FAT 20
SERVES FOUR, Cooking Time 1 hour

1 Heat the oil in a large pan and fry the onion in it until transparent.
2 Add courgettes and stir-fry for five minutes.
3 Wash lentils and add to pan. Add the water, garlic, lemon juice, cumin, basil, pepper and bay leaves.
4 Bring to the boil, cover and simmer for 35 minutes.
5 Cut potatoes into large chunks and add to pan, simmer for a further 25 minutes or until lentils and potatoes are cooked.

STUFFED POTATOES

YOU WILL NEED
4 large potatoes
1 lb (450 g) frozen
  sweetcorn, lightly cooked
  and cooled
½ tsp yeast extract
4 oz (100 g) mushrooms,
  chopped and fried in ½
  tbsp olive oil
2 tbsp skimmed milk
black pepper

1 Prepare potatoes for baking and bake in usual way for 60 minutes or until soft.
2 Split potatoes in half. Scoop out centres and mash with sweetcorn, mushrooms, yeast extract and pepper.
3 If the mixture is dry add the milk.
4 Pile the mixture back into the potatoes and heat under the grill for five minutes.

PROTEIN 45 CARBO 80 FAT 15
SERVES FOUR, Cooking Time 1 hour
5 minutes

CHESTNUT HOTPOT

Chestnuts are the lowest fat nuts by a long way, so enjoy yourself in chestnut season. Out of season you can use dried chestnuts which simply need soaking overnight.

YOU WILL NEED
5 oz (150 g) dried chestnuts
1 medium onion
8 oz (225 g) parsnips
8 oz (225 g) swede
8 oz (225 g) potato
8 oz (225 g) turnip
1 tsp bouillon powder
black pepper
1 oz (25 g) butter

1 Soak the chestnuts overnight.
2 Slice the onion and sauté in the butter in a large pan until soft.
3 Slice all the vegetables and add to the pot with the bouillion powder, pepper and chestnuts.
4 Simmer very gently until chestnuts are just soft, about 30 to 45 minutes.

PROTEIN 30 CARBO 55 FAT 45
SERVES FOUR, Cooking Time
45 minutes

BAKED BEANS ON TOAST

Most brands of baked beans are full of sugar. Whole Earth or Waitrose baked beans are not. They taste much better and are better for you.

YOU WILL NEED
2×14 oz (400 g) tins Whole
   Earth or Waitrose baked
   beans
4 slices wholemeal toast,
   lightly buttered

1 Heat baked beans as directed.
2 Serve on hot, lightly buttered toast.

PROTEIN 25 CARBO 40 FAT 20
SERVES FOUR

DESSERTS

APRICOT WHISK

This dessert tastes even better than it looks. Using dried apricots, rich in micronutrients, it can be made all year round.

YOU WILL NEED
8 oz (225 g) apricots
1/4 tsp natural vanilla essence
8 fl oz (225 ml) natural
   yoghurt
8 oz (225 g) Quark or low
   fat curd cheese
2 egg whites

1 Stew apricots until soft.
2 Liquidize with vanilla essence, yoghurt and curd cheese.
3 Whisk egg whites stiffly and fold into apricot mixture.
4 Cool in fridge before serving.

PROTEIN 85 CARBO 35 FAT 0
SERVES FOUR

RICE PUDDING

This good old-fashioned recipe simply uses brown instead of white rice for more fibre and taste.

YOU WILL NEED
4 oz (100 g) brown rice
2 oz (50 g) raisins
1½ pints (900 ml) skimmed
    milk
grated nutmeg
1 tsp honey

1 Put rice, raisins, milk and honey in an ovenproof dish.
2 Stir until honey is completely dissolved.
3 Sprinkle liberally with grated nutmeg.
4 Bake in an oven 150°C (300°F) gas mark 2 for two hours.

PROTEIN 85   CARBO 120   FAT 0
SERVES FOUR, Cooking Time 2 hours

RHUBARB AND BLACKCURRANT PIE

If you like rhubarb you'll love the combination of rhubarb and black-currant in this pie.

YOU WILL NEED
1 lb (450 g) rhubarb
8 oz (225 g) blackcurrants
½ tsp ground ginger
12 oz (350 g) Quark or low-fat curd cheese
¼ pint (150 ml) skimmed
    milk
1 tbsp honey
3 tbsp ground almonds

1 Stew rhubarb and blackcurrants until soft in a small amount of water.
2 Mix in ginger and put in ovenproof dish.
3 Mix curd cheese, milk and honey thoroughly.
4 Cover fruit with curd cheese mixture.
5 Sprinkle with almonds and lightly toast under a hot grill.

PROTEIN 80   CARBO 15   FAT 25
SERVES FOUR, Cooking Time 5–10 minutes

FRESH FRUIT SALAD

Adding one or two interesting fruits improves a fruit salad enormously, for example mango, kiwi, fresh lychee, strawberries, fresh dates or melon.

YOU WILL NEED
2 lb (900 g) mixed fruits
2 oz (50 g) dried apricots

PROTEIN 15   CARBO 55   FAT 0
SERVES FOUR

1 Cut fruit into cubes.
2 Stew apricots and liquidize, adding water to make into a pourable sauce.
3 Pour cooled sauce over fruit.

RASPBERRY SORBET

There are many variations to this theme, which allow you to pick fruit in season, freeze it and use it whenever you want. Just think, raspberries and strawberries all year round!

YOU WILL NEED
1 lb (450 g) raspberries
2 bananas, chopped into
   $1/_2$ inch lengths

PROTEIN 10   CARBO 20   FAT 0
SERVES FOUR

1 Freeze whole raspberries and chopped bananas.
2 Take out of the freezer and allow to partially thaw. About 5 minutes.
3 Liquidize or process in a food processor.
4 Serve immediately.

DATE STUFFED APPLES

The natural sugar in dates helps to sweeten the bitterest of cooking apples. Sprinkle with a little cinnamon and honey if you need it.

YOU WILL NEED
4 oz (100 g) dates
4 large cooking apples
1 tsp cinnamon
1 tbsp honey

PROTEIN 0   CARBO 55   FAT 0
SERVES FOUR, Cooking Time 1 hour

1 Chop dates roughly and core apples.
2 Stuff apple centres with dates and place in ovenproof dish.
3 Sprinkle with cinnamon and honey.
4 Pour water over apples to a depth of 1 inch in bottom of dish.
5 Bake in hot oven, 200°C (400°F) gas mark 6 for $^3/_4$ to 1 hour or until soft.

ALTERNATIVE DRINKS

Instead of drinking tea, try herb teas (Celestial Seasonings make some irresistible ones), or Rooibosch tea, which is best with milk. For real tea addicts, Luaka tea is lowest in tannin and caffeine.

Instead of coffee try dandelion coffee (Symington's or Dandex) or Barleycup. Decaffeinated coffee is second best – it still contains two other stimulants.

Drink at least half a pint of spring water a day – it tastes good, especially with ice and lemon.

Fruit juice is good, but check the label for added sugar. Dilute it with spring water.

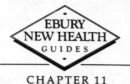

CHAPTER 11

WORK OUT YOUR OWN METABOLIC DIET

THE Batterham Diet Balancer is based on common sense. Using it, you can follow a low calorie diet, which is balanced for protein, carbohydrate and fat content. The problem with all calorie controlled diets today is that no matter what amount of calories per day are suggested the calories can be obtained from any source. Yet it is widely accepted that a well-balanced diet should be 15 per cent protein, 55 per cent carbohydrate and 30 per cent fat.

The Batterham Diet Balancer converts food content and calories into points, so that a food which has an equal number of Protein Points, Carbohydrate Points and Fat Points is a well-balanced food, as defined by the above criterion. It's simple. All you have to do is add up the points and if, at the end of the day, you have more fat points than the rest you've eaten too much fat. If you have more protein points than the rest, you've eaten more protein than you need. It is better to have the right number of points or less.

The one thing the Batterham Diet Balancer doesn't take into account is the vitamin, mineral and fibre content of foods. In the tables which follow, this important aspect of a food's quality, together with its overall balance, is represented by a ●●● rating. The highest star rating is ●●●●●. These foods are excellent all rounders. ●●●● foods are also good. No-star foods and ● foods should be avoided where possible.

Figures for protein, carbohydrate and fat are based on the easiest weight to be measured for a food. For example, that would be an egg or an apple. For foods which are usually measured in weight, 100 g (4 oz) is used. This is roughly equivalent to a tea-cup full, or small yoghurt pot full of grains, lentils, beans, nuts or seeds. All foods state the weight in grams and ounces on the package. Here is an example food:

Food and Description	Grams	Oz	Protein	Carbo	Fat	Rating
BREAD						
Wholemeal toast, ¼ oz butter	30	1	15	15	40	●●●

THE BATTERHAM DIET BALANCER TABLES

Foods are listed in alphabetical order. The more popular health food manufacturers' products are also listed alphabetically by company name.

Food and Description	Grams	Oz	Protein	Carbo	Fat	Rating
ALCOHOL (see drinks section)						
ALLINSONS PRODUCTS:						
bran biscuits	100	4	30	75	180	●
bran oatcakes	100	4	60	80	100	●●
coconut biscuits	100	4	40	60	230	●
fruit and nut biscuits	100	4	40	60	230	●
ginger biscuits	100	4	30	80	100	●●
honey biscuits	100	4	30	75	140	●
muesli biscuits	100	4	30	80	120	●●
oatmeal biscuits	100	4	40	70	195	●●
spice biscuits	100	4	30	75	130	●
walnut biscuits	100	4	45	70	145	●
wholemeal shortbread	100	4	35	85	155	●
bran bread mix	100	4	70	105	15	●●
malt bread mix	100	4	70	95	10	●●
white bread mix	100	4	70	105	10	●
wholewheat bread mix	100	4	70	95	15	●●●
honey bran	100	4	55	65	20	●●
bran plus	100	4	65	50	30	●●
broad bran	100	4	70	25	25	●●
wheatgerm (stabilized)	100	4	140	60	40	●●●
protose	100	4	15	120	60	●●
ravioli	100	4	15	20	10	●●●
rissolnut	100	4	65	100	105	●●
rolls (wheatmeal)	100	4	50	265	25	●●●
rolls (white)	100	4	55	265	25	●
sandwich spread	100	4	10	55	205	●
sausalatas	100	4	10	65	20	●
sausalene	100	4	15	110	50	●
sausfry	100	4	35	90	280	●
sauland	100	4	5	120	55	●
savoury cuts	100	4	5	90	0	●●●
savoury pudding	100	4	20	55	70	●
sunnybisks	100	4	100	70	10	●●

Food and Description	Grams	Oz	Protein	Carbo	Fat	Rating
tenderbits	100	4	5	85	0	
ALMONDS	55	2	50	5	185	●●●●
APPLE						
(1 medium)	115	4	0	15	0	●●●●
APRICOT						
(fresh)	85	3	5	10	0	●●●●
(dry)	30	1	5	15	0	●●●●
(canned)	115	4	5	45	0	●●●
ARTICHOKES						
(global)	115	4	5	5	0	●●●
ASPARAGUS						
(soft tips only)	115	4	10	0	0	●●●
AUBERGINE	115	4	5	5	0	●●●
AVOCADO PEAR	115	4	25	5	155	●●●
BACON						
(grilled 2 rashers)	55	2	75	0	120	●
(fried 2 rashers)	55	2	75	0	145	●
BANANA						
(weighed with skin)	170	6	5	25	5	●●●●
BARCELONA NUTS	55	2	35	5	220	●●●
BEANS						
(broad)	115	4	25	10	5	●●●●●
(butter)	115	4	45	25	5	●●●●●
(french)	115	4	5	0	0	●●●●●
(runner)	115	4	10	5	0	●●●●●
(baked in tomato sauce)	200	7	55	30	5	●●●
(haricot)	115	4	40	25	5	●●●●
(kidney – red)	115	4	45	25	5	●●●●
(mung – cooked dahl)	85	3	30	15	20	●●●●
(sprouts)	115	4	10	0	0	●●●●●
(soya beans)	100	4	15	50	25	●●
BEETROOT						
(pickled etc.)	30	1	5	5	0	●●
BEEF						
(steak fried)	115	4	175	0	100	●●●
(steak grilled)	115	4	165	0	85	●●●
(sirloin steak roast)	115	4	160	0	145	●●
(stewing steak)	85	3	140	0	55	●●●
(minced beef)	115	4	140	0	105	●●●

Food and Description	Grams	Oz	Protein	Carbo	Fat	Rating
(corned)	30	1	40	0	20	●
(canned stewing steak with gravy)	115	4	90	0	85	●
(burger fried)	55	2	60	5	60	●
(steak and kidney pie)	115	4	55	40	145	●●
(steak pudding)	115	4	65	30	85	●●
(stew)	115	4	115	10	105	●●
(curried)	115	4	60	15	70	●
(hotpot)	115	4	55	15	30	●●
(shepherds pie)	115	4	45	15	40	●●
BEMAX	7	1/4	10	5	5	
(crunchy)	100	4	75	85	20	●●●
BILBERRIES	115	4	5	20	0	●●●●
BISCUITS						
(chocolate)	30	1	10	25	50	●
(water)	30	1	15	30	20	●●
(cream crackers)	30	1	15	25	30	●●
(crispbread – rye)	30	1	15	30	5	●●●
(crispbread – wheat starch reduced)	30	1	70	15	15	●●●
(digestive – plain)	30	1	15	25	35	●●
(digestive – chocolate)	30	1	10	25	40	●
(ginger nuts)	30	1	10	30	25	●
(home-made)	30	1	10	25	40	●●
(oatcakes)	30	1	15	25	30	●●
(rich tea etc.)	30	1	10	30	30	●
(sandwich)	30	1	10	25	45	●●
(shortbread)	30	1	10	25	45	●
(shortcake)	30	1	10	25	40	●
(wafers – filled)	30	1	5	25	50	
BLACKBERRIES	115	4	10	10	0	●●●●
BLACKCURRANTS	115	4	5	10	0	●●●●●
BLACK PUDDING	30	1	20	5	40	●●
BLOATER						
(grilled)	30	1	25	0	20	●●●●
BOVRIL						
(and marmite/oxo/and bovril cubes)	7	1/4	15	0	0	●●
BRAIN						
(boiled)	85	3	55	0	50	●●●

Food and Description	Grams	Oz	Protein	Carbo	Fat	Rating
BRAN	7	¼	5	5	10	●●●
BRAZIL NUTS	55	2	35	5	210	●●●●
BREAD						
(currant)	55	2	20	40	10	●●
(hovis – thin slice)	30	1	15	20	5	●●●
(brown – thin slice)	30	1	15	15	5	●●●
(white – thin slice)	30	1	10	20	5	●
(white – fried)	30	1	15	25	75	
(white w. ⅛ oz butter)	30	1	10	20	20	
(white – toasted w. ¼ oz butter)	30	1	10	20	40	
(white w. ¼ oz butter and ½ oz jam/marmalade)	30	1	15	30	40	
(wholemeal – thin slice)	30	1	15	15	5	●●●
(wholemeal w. ⅛ oz butter)	30	1	15	15	20	●●●
(wholemeal – toasted w. ¼ oz butter)	30	1	15	15	40	●●●
(malt)	55	2	25	40	10	
(soda)	55	2	25	45	10	
(starch reduced)	30	1	65	20	5	●
(chapatis made with fat)	40	1½	20	30	35	
(chapatis – low fat)	40	1½	15	25	5	
BREAKFAST CEREALS						
(All Bran)	30	1	25	15	10	●●●
(Cornflakes)	30	1	15	35	5	●●
(Grapenuts)	30	1	15	30	5	●●
(Ready Brek)	30	1	20	25	15	●●
(Muesli – sugar free)	30	1	15	10	25	●●●
(Alpen)	30	1	20	10	25	●●
(Original Crunchy)	30	1	15	20	20	●●
(Puffed Wheat)	30	1	20	25	5	●
(Rice Krispies)	30	1	10	35	5	●
(Special K)	30	1	25	30	5	●●
(Sugar Puffs)	30	1	10	35	0	
(Weetabix)	30	1	20	35	5	●●●
BROCCOLI						
(tops – boiled)	115	4	20	5	0	●●●●
BRUSSELS SPROUTS	115	4	15	5	0	●●●●●
BUITONI PRODUCTS:						
high protein spaghetti	100	4	90	105	5	●●●

Food and Description	Grams	Oz	Protein	Carbo	Fat	Rating
other pasta	100	4	100	65	5	●●●
BUTTER	7	¹⁄₄	0	0	35	●
CABBAGE						
(and celeriac)	115	4	10	5	0	●●●●●
CAKES						
(currant buns)	115	4	45	85	50	●
(cheesecake)	115	4	25	35	230	●
(doughnuts)	115	4	35	75	110	●
(eclairs w. cream)	115	4	25	60	165	●
(fancy iced)	55	2	10	55	50	●
(fruit – rich)	115	4	25	90	75	●●
(fruit – iced – rich)	115	4	25	95	80	●
(fruit – plain)	115	4	30	90	90	●●
(gingerbread)	115	4	35	100	85	●●
(Madeira)	115	4	35	90	115	●●
(rock)	115	4	35	95	110	●●
(sponge – no fat)	115	4	60	85	45	●●
(sponge – jam filled)	115	4	25	100	35	●
CARROTS						
(fresh/canned)	115	4	5	5	0	●●●●●
CAULIFLOWER	115	4	10	0	0	●●●●
(cheese)	225	8	70	15	110	●●●
CELERY	115	4	5	5	0	●●●●
CHEESE						
(Camembert/Brie)	30	1	35	0	40	●●●
(Cheddar/Cheshire)	30	1	40	0	60	●●●
(Cottage)	115	4	85	5	5	●●●●
(Cream)	115	4	20	0	325	●●
(Danish Blue/Roquefort)	30	1	35	0	50	●●●
(Edam/Gouda/St. Paulin)	30	1	35	0	40	●●●
(Parmesan)	7	¹⁄₄	15	0	15	●●●
(processed)	30	1	35	0	45	●●
(pudding)	225	8	125	25	150	●
(soufflé)	115	4	70	15	130	●
(spread)	15	¹⁄₂	15	0	20	●
(Stilton)	30	1	40	0	70	●●
CHERRIES						
(fresh)	115	4	5	15	0	●●●●
(glacé)	30	1	0	20	0	●

Food and Description	Grams	Oz	Protein	Carbo	Fat	Rating
CHESTNUTS	55	2	5	30	10	●●●
CHICK-PEAS						
(raw)	55	2	60	40	20	●●●●
(cooked – dahl)	85	3	35	25	15	●●●●
CHICKEN						
(boiled)	115	4	175	0	50	●●●●
(fried)	115	4	150	0	100	●●●
(roast)	115	4	150	0	35	●●●
CHICORY	115	4	5	5	0	●●●●
COCKLES						
(and oysters)	30	1	15	0	0	●●●●
COCONUT						
(plain)	55	2	10	5	125	●●
(desiccated)	30	1	10	5	110	●
COD						
(and haddock/white fish						
poached or baked)	115	4	120	0	10	●●●●
(roe – fried)	30	1	30	0	20	●●●
CORNFLOUR	7	1/4	0	10	0	●
CORNISH PASTY	115	4	50	50	140	●
CRAB						
(boiled)	30	1	30	0	10	●●●
(canned)	30	1	30	0	0	●●
CRANBERRIES	115	4	5	5	0	●●●●
CREAM						
(double)	30	1	5	0	85	●
(single)	30	1	5	0	35	●●
(sterilized)	30	1	5	0	40	
(whipping)	30	1	5	0	60	
CUCUMBER	30	1	5	0	0	●●●●
CURRANTS						
(dried)	55	2	5	50	0	●●●
CURRY POWDER	7	1/4	5	5	5	●
CUSTARD						
(egg – home-made)	55	2	20	10	20	●●●
(made w. powder)	55	2	10	15	15	●
(tart)	115	4	35	45	115	●
DAMSONS	55	2	0	10	0	●●●●
DATES						
(dried)	55	2	5	50	0	●●●

Food and Description	Grams	Oz	Protein	Carbo	Fat	Rating
DIETADE PRODUCTS:						
conserves in fruit sugar	100	4	50	0	0	
fruits in fruit sugar	100	4	20	0	0	
fruits in water	100	4	5	0	0	
DRIPPING						
(beef, lard)	30	1	0	0	170	
DUCK						
(roast)	115	4	120	0	200	●●
EGGS						
(1 fried)	55	2	45	0	70	●●●
(1 scrambled/boiled/poached)	55	2	45	0	40	●●●●
(2 scrambled w. 1 oz milk and						
½ oz butter)	115	4	65	0	155	●●●
(omelette – plain made w. 2						
eggs)	115	4	65	0	115	●●●
(omelette – 1½ oz cheese)	155	5½	125	0	200	●●●
(omelette – 5 oz tomatoes)	255	9	70	5	115	●●●
(omelette – 2 rashers of bacon)	170	6	140	0	235	●
ENDIVE	30	1	5	0	0	●●●●
FATS						
(low fat spreads)	7	¼	0	0	20	●●●
FIGS						
(dried)	55	2	10	40	0	
FISH (separately listed)						
(white – fried in breadcrumbs)	115	4	110	5	95	●●
(white – fried in batter)	115	4	95	20	125	●●
(cakes – fried in breadcrumbs)	55	2	30	10	35	●
(fingers – fried in bread-						
crumbs)	30	1	20	5	15	●
(kedgeree)	115	4	80	15	50	●●
(paste)	30	1	25	0	20	●●
(pie)	115	4	45	20	40	●●
FLOUR						
(white – plain or S/R)	100	4	50	105	5	●
(white – bread-making)	100	4	60	100	5	●
FRUIT (listed separately)						
(pie-filling – canned)	115	4	0	40	0	●
(pie – individual)	115	4	25	90	105	●

Food and Description	Grams	Oz	Protein	Carbo	Fat	Rating
(pie – pastry top only)	115	4	10	45	50	●
(salad – canned)	115	4	0	40	0	●
GELATIN	30	1	130	0	0	●●●
GOLDEN SYRUP	30	1	0	30	0	
GOOSE						
(roast)	15	4	180	0	155	●●
GOOSEBERRIES						
(stewed w. sugar)	115	4	5	20	0	●●
GRANOSE PRODUCTS:						
bolognese sauce	100	4	10	30	0	●●
cannelloni	100	4	5	20	10	●●
chicken flavour pie filling	100	4	10	25	0	●●
chicken flavour pudding	100	4	20	40	45	●●
curry	100	4	20	30	0	●●
goulash	100	4	10	25	0	●●
granogen powder	100	4	65	110	125	●
granolac powder	100	4	65	85	155	●
natural bran	100	4	35	70	0	●●●
nutbrawn	100	4	20	45	85	●●
nuttolene	100	4	5	45	150	●
peanut butter	100	4	10	150	295	
GRAPEFRUIT						
(½ weighed w. skin)	200	7	5	5	0	●●●●
(canned)	115	4	5	25	0	●●●
GRAPES						
(and mangoes)	115	4	5	25	0	●●●●
GREENGAGES						
(raw)	55	2	5	20	0	●●●●
GREEN PEPPERS						
(raw or boiled)	30	1	0	0	0	●
GROUND GINGER	2	¹⁄₁₆	0	0	0	
GUAVAS						
(canned)	115	4	5	25	0	●●
HADDOCK	115	4	120	0	10	
HAM (boiled)	30	1	30	0	10	●●●
(chopped with pork)	30	1	20	0	40	●●
(collar joint – boiled)	115	4	125	0	185	●●
(gammon joint – boiled)	115	4	150	0	130	●●

Food and Description	Grams	Oz	Protein	Carbo	Fat	Rating
HAZELNUTS	55	2	25	5	125	●●●
HEART						
(ox – stewed)	85	3	145	0	30	●●●
(sheep's – roasted)	85	3	90	0	70	●●●
HERRING						
(fried)	30	1	35	0	25	●●●●
HONEY	30	1	0	30	0	●●
HORSERADISH	30	1	5	5	0	●
ITONA PRODUCTS:						
brown rice pudding	100	4	10	10	25	●●●●
hi fi biscuits	100	4	80	55	100	●
noots	100	4	35	210	160	●
noots bar	100	4	60	85	210	●
TVP minced beef	100	4	45	265	5	●
beef flavour chunks	100	4	45	265	5	●
ham flavour chunks	100	4	45	265	5	●
soya bean milk	100	4	5	20	70	●●●
tonabanga	100	4	50	85	0	●●
tonaburger	100	4	50	85	0	●●
tona 'c' food fish cake	100	4	50	85	0	●●
unflavoured mince	100	4	45	265	5	●●●
JAM (fruit/marmalade)	30	1	0	25	0	●
KIDNEY						
(stewed)	115	4	150	0	50	●●●
KIPPER						
(fillet)	30	1	30	0	20	●●●●
LAMB						
(chops)	115	4	110	0	155	●●●
(cutlets)	115	4	140	0	215	●●
(Irish stew)	115	4	30	15	45	●●●
(leg – roasted)	115	4	160	0	125	●●
(moussaka)	115	4	55	15	90	●●●
LAVERBREAD	30	1	5	0	5	●●●●
LEEKS	55	2	5	5	0	●●●●
LENTILS (cooked)	200	7	80	45	5	●●●●
(dahl)	200	7	50	30	40	●●●
LEMONS						
(and passion fruit)	55	2	5	5	0	●

Food and Description	Grams	Oz	Protein	Carbo	Fat	Rating
(curd – bought)	30	1	0	25	10	●
(curd – home-made)	30	1	5	15	25	●
LETTUCE	55	2	5	0	0	●●●●
LIVER	115	4	150	10	95	●●●●
LOBSTER						
(boiled)	30	1	35	0	5	●●●●
LOGANBERRIES						
(fresh)	115	4	5	5	0	●●●●●
(canned)	115	4	5	40	0	●●●
LYCHEES						
(canned)	115	4	5	30	0	●●●
MACARONI						
(dry weight)	115	4	85	125	15	●●●●
(cheese)	225	8	90	45	135	●●●
MACKEREL						
(fried)	30	1	35	0	20	●●●●
MANDARIN ORANGES						
(canned)	115	4	5	20	0	●●
MANGOES						
(canned)	115	4	0	30	0	●●
MARGARINE	100	4	0	0	490	
MARROW						
(boiled)	115	4	5	5	0	●●●
MARZIPAN	30	1	15	20	45	●
MEAT (listed separately)						
(paste)	30	1	25	0	20	●
MELON	200	7	5	10	0	●●●●
MILK						
(cow's/goat's)	30	1	5	5	10	●●●
(condensed – whole – sweetened)	30	1	15	20	15	●
(condensed – skimmed – sweetened)	30	1	15	25	0	●
(dried skimmed)	7	1/4	15	5	0	●●
(dried skimmed to make 1 pint)	55	2	110	40	5	●●
(evaporated – whole – unsweetened)	30	1	15	5	15	●
(whole – dried)	7	1/4	10	5	10	●●●
(whole dried to make 1 pint)	55	2	80	15	90	●●

Food and Description	Grams	Oz	Protein	Carbo	Fat	Rating
MINCEMEAT	30	1	0	25	5	●●●
MOLASSES	7	¼	0	10	0	
MUSHROOMS						
(boiled)	30	1	5	0	0	●●●
(fried)	55	2	5	0	65	●●
MUSSELS						
(and whelks/winkles)	30	1	25	0	5	●●●
NECTARINES	140	5	5	20	0	●●●●
OKRA	55	2	5	0	0	●●
OLIVES						
(in brine)	30	1	0	0	20	●
ONIONS						
(boiled)	30	1	0	0	0	●●●●
(fried)	30	1	5	5	55	●●●
(raw)	30	1	0	5	0	●●●●
(spring)	30	1	0	5	0	●●●
ORANGES	200	7	5	20	0	●●●●
OXTAIL						
(stewed)	85	3	140	0	70	●●●
PARSLEY	15	½	5	0	0	●●●
PARSNIPS	30	1	5	5	0	●●●
PARTRIDGE						
(roast)	85	3	170	0	40	●●●
PASTRIES						
(jam tarts)	30	1	5	25	25	●
(mince pies)	55	2	15	50	70	●
(scones – plain)	55	2	25	45	50	●●
(scotch pancakes/drop scones)	55	2	20	30	40	●●
PAW PAW						
(canned)	155	4	0	25	0	●●
PEACH						
(fresh)	140	5	5	15	0	●●●●
(canned)	115	4	0	35	0	●●
PEANUTS						
(fresh/salted)	55	2	75	5	170	●●
(butter)	30	1	35	5	95	●●
PEAR						
(fresh)	200	7	5	20	0	●●●●
(canned)	115	4	5	30	0	●●●

Food and Description	Grams	Oz	Protein	Carbo	Fat	Rating
PEAS						
(dried/boiled)	115	4	40	30	50	●●
(fresh/frozen)	115	4	35	10	5	●●●
(garden/canned)	115	4	30	10	5	●●●
(processed/canned)	115	4	40	20	5	●●●
(split/boiled)	115	4	50	35	5	●●●
PHEASANT						
(roast)	115	4	195	0	65	●●●
PICKLES etc.						
(apple chutney)	30	1	0	20	0	●●
(French dressing)	15	½	0	0	65	●●
(mayonnaise)	30	1	5	0	135	●
(piccalilli)	30	1	0	5	0	●
(salad cream)	30	1	5	5	45	●
(salad cream – low cal.)	30	1	5	5	15	●●
(sweet pickle)	30	1	0	15	0	●
(tomato chutney)	30	1	0	15	0	●
PIGEON						
(roast)	115	4	75	0	40	●●●
PILCHARDS						
(in tomato sauce)	30	1	30	0	10	●●●
PINEAPPLE						
(fresh)	115	4	5	20	0	●●●●
(canned)	115	4	0	30	0	●●
PIZZA						
(cheese and tomato)	225	8	115	75	160	●●
PLANTAIN						
(boiled)	30	1	0	10	0	●●
(fried)	30	1	5	20	15	●●
PLUMS	55	2	0	5	0	●●●
POMEGRANATE						
(juice)	55	2	0	10	0	●●
PORK						
(belly)	85	3	95	0	180	●●
(chops)	115	4	135	0	130	●●
(leg – roast)	115	4	165	0	135	●●
(luncheon meat)	30	1	20	5	45	●●●
(pie)	30	1	15	10	45	●●
PORRIDGE						
(made up)	200	7	15	20	10	●●●●

Food and Description	Grams	Oz	Protein	Carbo	Fat	Rating
POTATOES						
(baked in jacket – flesh only eaten)	200	7	20	55	0	●●●●
(boiled)	115	4	10	30	0	●●●
(chips – fried)	200	7	40	90	130	●
(crisps)	30	1	10	20	60	
(instant – powder – as served)	115	4	10	25	0	●
(mashed w. 1 oz milk + 1 oz butter per 1 lb)	115	4	10	30	40	●●
(roast)	85	3	15	30	25	
PRAWNS						
(boiled)	30	1	35	0	0	●●●
PREWITTS PRODUCTS:						
bran bread mix	100	4	85	70	15	●●●
brown bread mix	100	4	85	70	15	●●●
ever ready bread mix	100	4	95	65	15	●●
white bread mix	100	4	100	70	10	●
breakfast oats	100	4	90	70	40	●●●
natural wheat bran	100	4	25	70	25	●●●
oatmeal	100	4	90	70	40	●●●
porridge – wheatmeal	100	4	105	50	5	●●●●
rye flour	100	4	95	80	15	●●●●
unpolished rice	100	4	105	40	15	●●●
wheat embryo	100	4	60	140	40	●●●
bran muesli	100	4	65	55	55	●●●●
golden grains	100	4	90	55	55	●●●
honey muesli	100	4	90	55	50	●●●
muesli	100	4	90	60	35	●●●●
muesli – deluxe	100	4	85	55	80	●●●●
wholewheat flakes	100	4	110	50	20	●●●●
FRUIT BARS:						
apple and date	100	4	75	20	10	●●●
banana	100	4	80	15	5	●●●
date and fig	100	4	85	15	10	●●●
fruit and bran	100	4	75	25	25	●●●
fruit and nut	100	4	75	80	55	●●●
muesli	100	4	70	30	55	●●●
Brazilian mix	100	4	50	150	105	●●
5-cereal savoury mix	100	4	60	120	55	●●
rissole mix	100	4	55	145	105	●●

Food and Description	Grams	Oz	Protein	Carbo	Fat	Rating
earth wonder mixes (av)	100		80	65	60	●●
PRUNES						
(dried)	55	2	5	30	0	●●
PUDDINGS						
(apple crumble)	225	8	20	115	95	●●●
(bread and butter)	225	8	75	55	110	●●●
(ice cream)	55	2	10	20	25	●●
(jelly cubes – 1)	15	½	5	10	0	●
(jelly made w. water)	115	4	10	20	0	●
(jelly made w. milk)	115	4	15	25	10	●●
(lemon meringue pie)	115	4	25	70	100	●
(meringues – no cream)	55	2	15	75	0	●
(milk puddings e.g. rice)	200	7	45	55	50	●●●
(rice pudding – canned)	200	7	35	40	30	●●
(pancakes)	200	7	70	70	200	●●
(Queen of puddings)	170	6	45	80	80	●●
(sponge – steamed)	115	4	35	70	115	●●
(suet – steamed)	115	4	25	65	125	●
(treacle tart)	115	4	25	95	95	●
(trifle)	170	6	30	55	65	●
(Yorkshire)	115	4	40	40	70	●●
PUMPKIN						
(raw)	115	4	5	5	0	●●●●
QUARK	100	4	75	2	5	●●●
QUICHE LORRAINE	115	4	90	35	195	●
QUINCES						
(flesh only)	115	4	0	10	0	●●●●
RABBIT						
(STEWED)	115	4	150	0	45	●●●
RADISHES	30	1	0	0	0	●●●●
RAISINS						
(dried and sultanas)	55	2	5	50	0	●●●
RASPBERRIES						
(fresh)	55	2	5	5	0	●●●●
(canned)	115	4	5	35	0	●●
RHUBARB						
(stewed – no sugar)	115	4	5	0	0	●●●
(stewed w. sugar)	115	4	5	20	0	●●

Food and Description	Grams	Oz	Protein	Carbo	Fat	Rating
RICE						
(dry)	30	1	10	35	0	●●●●
(boiled)	115	4	15	45	5	●●●●
SALAD DRESSING	100		0	5	200	●
(herb dressing)	100		0	5	240	●
SALMON						
(canned)	30	1	30	0	15	●●●
(smoked)	30	1	40	0	15	●●●
SARDINES						
(canned in oil)	30	1	35	0	25	●●●
(canned in tomato sauce)	30	1	25	0	20	●●●
SAUCES						
(Bolognese)	55	2	25	5	40	●●
(bread)	30	1	5	5	10	●●●
(brown)	15	½	0	5	0	●●
(cheese)	30	1	15	5	25	●●●
(tomato – sauce)	15	½	0	0	5	●●●●
(tomato – purée)	30	1	10	5	0	●●●●
(tomato – ketchup)	15	½	0	10	0	●●
(white – savoury)	30	1	5	5	20	●●
(white – sweet)	30	1	5	10	15	●●
SAUSAGES						
(beef – 1 sausage)	55	2	40	10	60	
(Frankfurter – 1)	30	1	15	0	45	
(pork – 1 sausage)	55	2	40	10	85	
(roll)	30	1	10	15	55	
(salami)	30	1	30	0	80	
(saveloy)	55	2	30	10	70	
SCALLOPS						
(boiled)	30	1	35	0	5	●●●
SCAMPI						
(fried in breadcrumbs)	30	1	20	10	30	●●
SEAKALE	55	2	5	0	0	●●●●
SEMOLINA						
(dry)	30	1	15	30	5	●●●
SESAME SEEDS	30	1	35	80	10	●●●
SHRIMPS						
(boiled)	30	1	35	0	5	●●●

Food and Description	Grams	Oz	Protein	Carbo	Fat	Rating
SOUPS						
(cream of chicken)	280	10	25	20	45	●●●
(cream of chicken – condensed)	140	5	20	10	60	●●
(chicken noodle)	280	10	10	15	5	●
(lentil – home made)	280	10	65	45	65	●●●●
(minestrone)	280	10	10	15	10	●●
(mushroom)	280	10	15	15	45	●●
(oxtail)	280	10	35	20	30	●
(oxtail)	280	10	20	15	15	●●
(tomato – cream of)	280	10	10	25	55	●●
(tomato – condensed)	140	5	15	30	60	●
(tomato)	280	10	10	25	10	●●●
(vegetable)	280	10	25	25	10	●●●●
SOYA FLOUR						
(low fat)	30	1	70	10	15	●●●●
(full fat)	30	1	55	10	40	●●●
SOYA MILK	100	4	5	20	70	●●
SPAGHETTI						
(dry)	115	4	85	130	5	●●
(canned in tomato sauce)	200	7	20	35	10	●
SPINACH	115	4	15	5	5	●●●●●
SPRATS						
(fried)	30	1	40	0	65	●●●
SPRING GREENS	115	4	10	0	0	●●●●●
STRAWBERRIES						
(canned)	115	4	5	35	0	●●
(fresh)	115	4	5	10	0	●●●●
SUGAR						
(demerara)	7	¼	0	10	0	
(white)	7	¼	0	10	0	
SUNFLOWER SEEDS	30	1	35	80	10	●●●
SWEDES	115	4	5	5	0	●●●●
SWEETCORN						
(canned)	115	4	20	25	5	●●●●
(on the cob)	115	4	25	35	15	●●●●
SWEET POTATOES	115	4	5	30	5	●●●●●
SWEETS						
(boiled)	30	1	0	35	0	
(Bounty bar)	30	1	5	25	45	

Food and Description	Grams	Oz	Protein	Carbo	Fat	Rating
(chocolate – milk)	30	1	15	25	50	
(chocolate – plain)	30	1	5	25	50	
(chocolate – filled)	30	1	5	25	50	
(fruit gums)	30	1	0	20	0	
(Liquorice Allsorts)	30	1	5	30	5	
(Mars bar)	30	1	10	25	35	
(pastilles)	30	1	10	25	0	
(peppermints)	30	1	0	40	0	
(toffees)	30	1	5	30	30	
TANGERINES	85	3	5	5	0	●●●●
TAPIOCA						
(raw)	30	1	0	35	0	●●●
TOFU	100	4	40	25	4	●●●●
TOMATOES						
(raw)	85	3	5	5	0	●●●●
(fried – 1)	70	2½	5	5	25	●●
TONGUE						
(stewed or boiled)	85	3	80	0	125	●
TRIPE						
(stewed)	55	2	45	0	15	●
TROUT						
(smoked or stewed)	30	1	25	0	5	●●●
TUNA						
(canned in brine)	30	1	35	0	25	●●●
(canned in oil)	30	1	35	0	40	●●
TURKEY						
(roast)	115	4	175	0	20	●●●
TURNIP	115	4	5	5	5	●●●●
(tops)	55	2	10	0	0	●●●●
VENISON						
(roast)	85	3	160	0	10	●●●
VINEGAR	15	½	0	0	0	●●
WATERCRESS	30	1	5	0	0	●●●●●
YAMS	115	4	10	45	0	●●●●
YOGHURT	30	1	5	5	5	●

DRINKS – LISTED IN ALPHABETICAL ORDER (EXCLUDING ALCOHOL)

	ml	fl oz	Protein	Carbo	Fat	Rating
APPLE JUICE	115	4	0	20	0	●●●●
BOURNVITA	7	$\frac{1}{4}$	5	10	5	
CHOCOLATE (drinking)	7	$\frac{1}{4}$	5	10	5	
COCA COLA	225	8	0	35	0	
COCOA (powder)	7	$\frac{1}{4}$	5	0	10	
COFFEE (Camp with chicory)	7	$\frac{1}{4}$	0	5	0	
(ground roast)	200	7	5	0	0	
(instant)	4	$\frac{1}{8}$	5	0	0	
GRAPEFRUIT JUICE (sweetened)	115	4	5	15	0	●
(unsweetened)	115	4	0	10	0	●●●
HORLICKS	7	$\frac{1}{4}$	5	5	5	●
LEMONADE	225	8	0	20	0	
LEMON JUICE (and soda water)	30	1	0	0	0	●●●
LIME CORDIAL (undiluted)	30	1	0	10	0	
LUCOZADE	225	8	0	55	0	
MILK (see listing under food)						
ORANGE (juice – sweetened)	115	4	5	20	0	
(juice – unsweetened)	115	4	5	15	0	●●●●
(squash – undiluted)	30	1	0	10	0	
OVALTINE	7	$\frac{1}{4}$	5	10	0	●
PINEAPPLE JUICE	115	4	5	20	0	●●●●
ROSEHIP SYRUP	30	1	0	25	0	●
RIBENA (undiluted)	30	1	0	25	0	●
TEA (without milk/sugar)	200	7	0	0	0	●●
TOMATO JUICE	115	4	5	5	0	●●●●

Alcoholic Beverages	ml	fl oz	Carbo
Brown Ale (bottled)	300	½ pint	30
Lager small (bottled)	300	½ pint	30
Bitter small can	300	½ pint	30
Pale Ale (bottled)	300	½ pint	30
Draught Bitter & Dry Cider	300	½ pint	30
Draught Mild	300	½ pint	25
Lager (canned)	550	15½	50
Stout Mackeson etc. small	300	½ pint	40
Stout Extra e.g. Guinness	300	½ pint	40
Strong Ale e.g. Barley Wine etc. small (bottled)	300	½ pint	75
Sweet Cider small (bottled)	300	½ pint	45
Vintage Cider small (bottled)	300	½ pint	100
Red Wine per glass e.g. Beaujolais, Burgundy & Rose	60	2½	20
Dry White Wine (per glass)	60	2½	15
Medium Dry Wine (per glass)	60	2½	20
Sweet White Wine (per glass)	60	2½	25
Sparkling White Wine per glass	60	2½	20
Port & Sweet Sherry & Vermouth Martini etc. sweet (per measure)		⅓ gill	20
Dry Sherry & Medium Sherry & Dry Vermouth & Martini (per measure)		⅓ gill	20
Cherry Brandy (per measure)		⅙ gill	20
Curaçao (per measure)		⅙ gill	25
Spirits, 70% proof (per measure)		⅙ gill	20

Please note that it is not a bonus to raise your carbohydrate score by drinking alcohol. This is the wrong form of carbohydrate being allied to sugar. It is assumed that no more than 3 glasses of wine or equivalent a week is drunk.

HOW TO WORK OUT YOUR OWN POINTS FOR NEW FOODS

Not all foods are listed in the previous pages. But as long as you have values for the fat, protein and carbohydrate content of any food, together with the total calories of the food, you can work out the points yourself.

The Batterham Diet Balancer is based upon a diet containing 15 per cent protein, 55 per cent carbohydrate and 30 per cent fat. Here's an example, which explains how the points are allocated. If you have a day's menu which provides 2,500 calories and is balanced to the above percentages of protein, carbohydrate and fat then:

─────────────────────── **Protein** ───────────────────────
15% × 2,500 = 375 kcal – the calories provided from protein
As protein provides 4 kcal per gram
375/4 = 94 G – THE AMOUNT OF PROTEIN

────────────────────── **Carbohydrate** ──────────────────────
55% × 2,500 = 1,375 kcal – the calories provided by carbohydrate
As carbohydrate provides 3.75 kcal per gram
1,375/3.75 = 367 G OF CARBOHYDRATE

────────────────────────── **Fat** ──────────────────────────
30% × 2,500 = 750 kcal – the calories provided from fat
As fat provides 9 kcal per gram
750/9 = 83 G – THE AMOUNT OF FAT

The Batterham Diet Balancer allocates points for each calorie equivalent gram of food.

94 g of protein   = 500 PROTEIN POINTS
367 g of carbo   = 500 CARBO POINTS
83 g of fat   = 500 FAT POINTS
So a balanced 500 points diet = 2,500 CALORIES
So a balanced 400 points diet = 2,000 CALORIES
So a balanced 350 points diet = 1,750 CALORIES
So a balanced 300 points diet = 1,500 CALORIES
So a balanced 250 points diet = 1,250 CALORIES

HERE'S HOW TO WORK OUT YOUR NEW FOOD

If you want to work out the points for an imaginary food you need to know three things. The protein content (called 'A'), the carbohydrate content (called 'B'), the fat content (called 'C') and the calories provided by the food (called 'D').

A/94 × 500 × D/2,500 = PROTEIN POINTS
B/367 × 500 × D/2,500 = CARBOHYDRATE POINTS
C/83 × 500 × D/2,500 = FAT POINTS

Simpler still is this equation:
A × D × 0.0021 = PROTEIN POINTS
B × D × 0.00054 = CARBOHYDRATE POINTS
C × D × 0.0024 = FAT POINTS

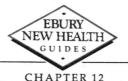
CHAPTER 12

BINGEING – THE ALLERGY CONNECTION

THE word allergy often provokes connotations beyond its original meaning. An allergy to a particular substance simply means an intolerance that causes a reaction in the immune system. We all have minor intolerances to coffee and alcohol, for example, which alter biochemical functions. More pronounced allergies can be responsible for more pronounced mental and physical symptoms. These symptoms include mood changes, like depression, as well as water retention, increased appetite, sleepiness after meals, mental fatigue and a host of other minor ailments. But what have allergies got to do with weight loss?

If you are allergic to a particular food, you are likely to crave that food and therefore eat it frequently. It's as if you are mildly addicted. Through working with a number of allergic and overweight clients, it became clear that bingeing, or uncontrolled overeating, often happened only with certain food groups. When clients were instructed to eat as much as they liked of anything but not the suspected allergen (food that provokes an allergic reaction), bingeing often ceased completely. When the allergen was totally avoided clients sometimes lost as much as 7 lb weight overnight. This sort of short-term weight loss had to be the result of excess fluid retention and nothing to do with fat.

One of the physical symptoms of an allergic reaction can be sudden fluctuations in blood sugar level. This in turn affects appetite. Could it be that the initial allergic reaction to the food was setting the scene for increased appetite and hence bingeing? In honesty, nobody has a definite answer to this question, but my observations with a number of clients certainly show that sometimes allergies do play a role in overweight problems.

The most common food groups that people are allergic to are:

1 Grains

Grains include wheat, oats, maize, barley, rye and even rice. Few people react to all of these, and wheat is by far the most common allergen.

2 Milk

Milk products include milk, cheese, butter and yoghurt. However, it is a particular protein in milk that causes offence and since there is little protein in butter this doesn't usually cause a reaction. Yoghurt and cheese can also sometimes be tolerated by the milk allergic. Some can tolerate goat's milk but not cow's.

3 Eggs

Egg allergy is quite common. Surprisingly, those that react to chicken's eggs rarely react to chicken or eggs from different birds, like duck eggs.

4 Pip/Nuts

The pip/nut family includes fruits with pips, nuts, including chocolate, derived from cocoa, and coffee. It is rare that the 'pip/nut' allergic reacts to all fruits and nut derivatives, but if you know you react to some nuts, be wary of other members of this group.

5 Sugar

Sugar can cause symptoms because of blood sugar fluctuations, which aren't necessarily allergically mediated. But for some people, sugar also causes an allergic response. Sometimes only certain forms of sugar cause a reaction. Those that are corn allergic often react to corn sugar, but not to other forms.

6 Food Additives/Preservatives

A number of food colourings and preservatives have been identified as causing allergic reactions. Particularly powerful seems to be the colourings called A20 dyes which are most of the E numbers between E102 and E180. These are best avoided anyway.

HOW TO TEST FOR FOOD ALLERGIES

If you suspect that you may be allergic here is a simple way to test. It is not fool-proof but it is a good way to investigate the possibility. First of all, list all those foods that you would find hardest to give up, that you eat once or twice almost every day, that you suspect may make you feel worse or affect your appetite. Write these down below.

1_____

2_____

3_____

4_____

5_____

Avoid all these substances strictly for 28 days. And do check the contents of the foods you eat carefully to see whether they contain any of the above. It is best to prepare yourself well by stocking up with your allergen-free foods before starting.

If you are avoiding WHEAT stay off all bread, cakes, biscuits, pasta, sauces, cereals etc. Alternatives are oat cakes, rice cakes, rye crisp-bread, sauces made with corn flour, corn or oat based cereals and pastry made with corn and almond meal instead of wheat.

If you are avoiding MILK stay off all milk, cheese, yoghurt, butter, chocolate and foods containing milk produce. Good alternatives are soya milk, or nut cream, made by blending nuts with water (cashews are particularly good). Drink herb teas that do not require milk, and have more free range eggs if cheese is a major source of your protein.

Then do this Simple Pulse Test.

1 Take your pulse at rest (after five minutes sitting down), for 60 seconds. Your pulse can be found inside the bony protuberance on the thumb side of your wrist.

2 Then eat more than usual of the No. 1 food.

3 Take your pulse after 10, 30 and 60 minutes. Make sure you take your pulse at rest for the duration of 60 seconds.

4 Keep a record of any symptoms over the next 24 hours.

If your pulse increases by ten points or if you have any noticeable symptoms within 24 hours, avoid this substance and wait 24 hours before testing the next item on your list.

If your pulse does not increase by ten points and you have no change in symptoms, reintroduce this food (in moderation) into your diet and proceed with the same test for food No. 2.

You will find a form for keeping a record of your pulse symptoms on the next page. By avoiding foods which raise your pulse or cause symptoms you will probably find improvements in your health. The Metabolic Diet and supplements will also help to further reduce your allergic potential. After two to three months you may then find that you can tolerate small, infrequent amounts of the allergen. For some people the allergy disappears completely. Others have to be careful about certain foods for life. Once you have more than a sneaking suspicion that you are allergic it is best to see a nutritionist, who can help you further.

USEFUL ADDRESSES

Asset is the National Association for Health and Exercise Teachers. All fully accredited exercise teachers should be members, so you can contact this organization to find out about good teachers in your area. Their address is 202 The Avenue, Kennington, Oxford OX1 5RN. Tel: 0865 736066.

The Fitness Centre in central London can assess your fitness level and advise on the best form of aerobic exercise for you. The Fitness Centre has many different aerobics, dance and circuit training classes. The Fitness Centre, 11 Floral Street, Covent Garden, London WC2.

Health + Plus vitamin company supply vitamin and mineral supplements, including Glucomannan, by mail order. Ring or write to Health + Plus, Health + Plus House, 118 Station Road, Chinnor, Oxon. Tel: 0844 52098.

Institute for Optimum Nutrition offers courses and personal consultations with trained nutritionists, including Patrick Holford. They can assess your fat percentage and devise an individually tailored nutrition programme to assist with weight loss and general health improvement. A directory of ION-trained nutritionists is available on request. To receive ION's information pack please ring or write to ION, 5 Jerdan Place, London SW6 1BE. Tel: 01 385 7984.

RECOMMENDED READING

The following books will help you to dig deeper into nutrition and weight loss.

Patrick Holford – *Vitamin Vitality* (Collins) 1985. A thoroughly researched book which establishes why so many people are sub-optimally nourished and how to work out your own vitamin and mineral needs for optimum health.

ION Survey (ION Publications) 1984. A well-documented follow-up of 100 people on 'optimum nutrition' over one year, including the results achieved with overweight clients. (Only available direct from ION, price £1.)

Patrick Holford – *Whole Health Manual* (Thorsons) 1983. A clear and concise introduction to the basic principles of nutrition, explaining how your body works, how to balance your diet, and how to use vitamins and minerals.

Dr Theron Randolph – *Allergies: Your Hidden Enemy* (Thorsons). An excellent introduction to food allergy, what it is and how to reduce your allergic potential.

Suzie Orbach – *Fat is a Feminist Issue* (Penguin). Why do we overeat and why are we sometimes obsessed with thinness? This book explores some of the psychological pressures tied up with weight loss.

Geoffrey Cannon – *Dieting Makes You Fat* (Sphere) 1984. This book presents clear evidence that crash dieting doesn't work, and that raising metabolic weight is the only answer to long-term weight control.

Covert Bailey – *Fit or Fat?* (Sphere) 1980. One of the first, and one of the best, books explaining the connection between exercise, metabolism and weight loss.

Dr Kenneth Cooper – *The Aerobics Way* (Corgi) 1978. Cooper is sometimes called the father of aerobics and his book helps you to get fit quickly and safely.

REFERENCES

A list of key 'metabolic' references is available from the author. Please send £1 and a self-addressed envelope to Patrick Holford, The Institute for Optimum Nutrition, 5 Jerdan Place, London SW6 1BE.

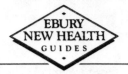

INDEX

Absorption of nutrients, 22–3
Additives, food, 22, 35, 38
  allergy to, 122
Adrenaline, 18–19
Aerobic exercise, 45–6, 50, 51, 52, 53
Alcohol consumption, effects of, 23, 27, 37, 38, 59
Alfalfa sprouts: recipes, 80, 81
  saponins in, 33
Allergy: definition, 121
  food groups causing, 121–2
  symptoms, 121
  to test for, 122–3
Almonds see Nuts
Amino acids, 14, 29
Anti-nutrients, 22
Appetite, regulating, 19
Apples: effect on blood sugar, 36
  pectin content, 32
  recipes, 75, 99
Apricot whisk, 96
Ascorbate, 25

Badminton, 53, 55
Bananas: effect on blood sugar, 36
  pectin content, 32
  potassium content, 31
  recipes, 76, 84, 98
Basketball, 55
Batterham Diet Balancer, 26, 27–8, 73, 100
  tables, 101–19
  to work out new foods, 119–20
Beans, 16, 31
  baked, on toast, 28, 96
  effect on blood sugar, 36
  polyphenols in, 33
  recipe, 85
Biscuits: effect on blood sugar, 36
BLISSS exercise programme, 7, 49, 57
Blood sugar level: and appetite, 19
  balancing, 16–17, 27, 34–7
Breakfast recipes, 75–8

Caffeine, 38
Calcium: absorption of, 22

optimum daily level, 25
Calories: counting, 9, 10
  definition, 10
  empty, 29
  used in exercise, 45–6
Carbohydrates, 6, 7, 14, 16, 27
  low carbohydrate diets, 12
  in refined form, 33, 43
Carrots: effect on blood sugar, 36, 37
  pectin content, 32
  recipes, 79, 82, 84, 88
Cellulose, 16, 26
Cereals: effect on blood sugar, 36
Chestnut hotpot, 95
Chicken, 30, 31
  salad, 91
Chick peas: recipes, 83, 94
Chocolate, 38
  allergy to, 122
Cholesterol, reducing: and Glucomannan, 42, 43
  and saponins, 33
  and vitamins B3 and C 24
Choline: optimum daily level, 25
Chromium: deficiency, 17, 24
  and formation of GTF, 34
  loss in refined food, 28
  optimum daily level, 25
  and weight control, 24
Cigarettes see Smoking
Circuit weight training, 52, 53, 54–5
Cobalamine, 25
Coffee, 23, 38
  dandelion, 99
  decaffeinated, 35, 38, 99
  excess, 18, 27
Cola drinks, 38
Colourings, food, 38
  allergy to, 122
Constipation: and Glucomannan, 43–4
Corn: recipes, 87, 95
Corticosteroids, 19
Cottage cheese and alfalfa sandwich, 81
Courgettes: recipes, 89, 94
Couscous, spicy almond, 91
Cycling, 46, 53, 54

Dairy products: allergy to, 122
  effect on blood sugar, 36
Dance exercises, 51, 53
Date stuffed apples, 99
Dessert recipes, 96–9
Dextrose, 16
Diabetes, 15, 17, 33
  and Glucomannan fibre, 42–3
  and obesity, 43
Drinks, stimulant, 18, 23, 39, 59
  alternatives to, 99
Drugs, effects of, 23

Eggs, 27, 30, 31
  allergy to, 122
Energy: how food converts to, 14, 15
  monitoring, 74
Enzymes, 14, 16, 22
Exercise: and appetite, 48
  calories used in, 10, 45–6
  and metabolic rate, 48–9, 57
  monitoring, 72, 73
  and nutritional needs, 23
  principles to follow, 49–50
  stamina-developing, 51
  starting programme, 49, 57
  strength-promoting, 51–2
  for suppleness, 52–3
  ways to increase, 47
  and weight loss, 45–8

Fasting, 13
Fat, 14, 15
  high-fat diets, 12
  risks from excess, 27
Fatty acids, essential, 15
Fertilizers, use of, 28
Fibre, 12
  high-fibre diets, 11–12, 26–7, 40
  sources of, 12
  see also Glucomannan fibre
Fibre, 'gum', 32–3
Fish, 30, 32
  recipes, 89, 90
Flour: refined, 28, 30
  wholewheat, 22, 30
Folic acid: optimum daily level, 25
Football, 53, 55

Fructose, 16, 33, 37
Fruit, 31 (*see* Apples *etc*)
  effect on blood sugar, 36, 37
  recipes, 77, 84, 98
Frying food, 59

Gardening, 53
Glucagon, 19
Glucomannan fibre, 7, 32–3
  and constipation relief, 43–4
  and diabetes, 42–3
  and glucose intolerance, 43
  and heart disease, 42
  how and when to take, 44,
    69–70
  source, 40
  tests on, 40–1
Glucose, 14, 16, 18, 33, 37
  intolerance to, 17, 18, 19, 34–5,
    43
Glucose Tolerance Factor (GTF),
  24, 34
Glycaemic index of common
  foods, 36–7
Golf, 53
Grains, 16
  allergy to, 121
  effect on blood sugar, 36
GTF *see* Glucose Tolerance Factor
Guar gum, 32–3, 43

Hamburgers, 30
Heart disease, 15, 27
  and Glucomannan fibre, 42
  and pulse rate, 55
  and saponins, 33
Hiatus hernia, 51
Housework: and fitness, 46–7
Hummus, 83
Hyperglycaemia, 33, 34, 43
Hypoglycaemia, 17, 33, 34, 43

Inositol: optimum daily level, 25
Insulin, 17, 19, 28, 33
Iron: optimum daily level, 25
Island dressing, 85

Jogging, 45–6, 49, 53–4

Kedgeree, 90
Ketones, 12
Kidney disease, 15, 27
Konjac plant, 40

Lactose, 16
Lentils, 16, 31
  effect on blood sugar, 36
  recipes, 81, 92, 94
Lettuce, 31
Lunch recipes, packed, 79–81

Magnesium: optimum daily level,
  25
Maltose, 16, 37
Manganese: deficiency, 22

optimum daily level, 25
  loss in refined food, 28
  peas as source, 31
Metabolic diet, 7–8
  do's and don'ts, 58, 59
  menus for 15 days, 60–7
  shopping list for, 67–8
  working out your own, 100-20
Metabolic rate: and dieting, 8
  to increase, 6–7, 14, 48–9, 57, 59
Metabolism: definition, 6
Milk: allergy to, 122
  effect on blood sugar, 36
Minerals, 19, 20
  deficiencies in, 22
  optimum daily level, 25
  taking supplements, 69, 70
  see also Nutrients
Muesli, apple, 75
Muscles: strengthening, 51–2
  stretching, 52
  turning to fat, 46
Mushrooms, 31
  recipe, 93

Niacinamide, 25
Nicotinic acid, 24
Nutrients, 20, 21
  absorption of, 22–3
  and anti-nutrients, 22
  deficiencies, 22
  needs and biochemistry, 21 2
  needs and heredity, 21
Nuts, 31
  allergy to, 122
  recipes, 76, 78, 82, 87, 91, 95
  saponins in, 33

Obesity: and diabetes, 43
Oils, cooking, 58
Oranges: effect on blood sugar,
  36
  lack of vitamin C in, 28

Pantothenate, 25
Pantothenic acid, 23
Pear and cashew yoghurt, 76
Peas: effect on blood sugar, 37
  manganese content, 31
Pectin, 32
Peppers, stuffed, 92
Phytates, 22
Polyphenols, 33
Polysaccharides, 16
Porridge, Scots, 78
Potassium: bananas as source, 31
Potatoes, 16, 31, 32
  effect on blood sugar, 36, 37
  recipes, 79, 80, 95
Preservatives, food, 122
Protein, 6, 14
  high-protein diets, 12–13
Prune and almond yoghurt, 78
Psychocallisthenics, 53

Pulse rate: and exercise, 51, 55–6
  testing for allergy, 123
Pulses: effect on blood sugar, 36,
  37
Pyridoxine, 25

Raspberry sorbet, 98
Retinol, 25
Rhubarb and blackcurrant pie, 97
Riboflavin, 25
Rice: effect on blood sugar, 36
  and loss of nutrients, 28
  recipes, 93, 97
Running, 45, 46, 51, 53–4

Salad recipes, 79, 83, 84–7, 91
Salt, 23
  excess consumption, 39
Saponins, 33
Sausages, 30
Selenium deficiency, 22
Skiing, 53
Skipping, 51, 53, 54
Slimming pills, 6, 11, 13, 40–1
Smoking, effects of, 38
Sodium, excess, 39
Soup recipes, 81–2
Spaghetti napolitana, 90
Spinach, 28–9, 31
  recipe, 85
Squash, 46, 53, 55
Starch, 16
Starch blocker tablets, 13
Starters, recipes for, 81–4
Stress: effects of, 18–19, 35
  and need for nutrients, 23
Sucrose, 16, 37
Sugar: allergy to, 122
  effect on blood sugar, 37
  refined, 28
Swimming, 45–6, 51, 53, 54

Tabouli, 93
Tannic acid, 39
Tartrazine, effects of, 38
Tea: cutting consumption, 59
  effects of, 23, 39
  excess, 18
  herb, 59, 99
Tennis, 46, 53, 54
Theobromine, 38, 39
Thiamine, 25
Tocopherol, d-alpha, 25
Tofu and alfalfa sandwich, 80
Tomatoes, 31, 32
  recipes, 83, 87
Tuna and chick pea feast, 94

Vegetables, 16, 31
  cooking, 58
  effect on blood sugar, 36, 37
  recipes, 82, 84, 88
  see also Carrots *etc*
Vitamins, 7, 19, 20, 26

optimum daily levels, 25
  and weight loss, 23–4
  see also Nutrients
Vitamin supplements, 7, 25, 69
  best makes, 70
  daily programme, 69, 70

Walking, 47–8, 51, 53, 55

Watercress salad, 86
Weight: ideal (for height), 71, 72
  monitoring, 71
Weight lifting, 50
Wheat: loss of nutrients, 28
  and zinc absorption, 22

Yoga, 50, 52

Yoghurt: allergy to, 122
  effect on blood sugar, 36
  recipes, 76

Zinc: deficiency, 21, 22, 25
  loss in refined food, 28
  optimum daily level, 25